Current Clinical Strategies

Manual of HIV/AIDS Therapy

2001 Edition

Douglas C. Princeton, M.D.

Current Clinical Strategies Publishing

www.ccspublishing.com

Digital Book and Updates

Purchasers of this book may download the digital book and updates of this text at the Current Clinical Strategies Publishing internet site: www.ccspublishing.com.

Copyright © 2001 Current Clinical Strategies Publishing Inc. All rights reserved. This book, or any parts thereof, may not be reproduced or stored in an information retrieval network without the permission of the Publisher. The reader is advised to consult other references and the package insert before using any therapeutic agent. The publisher disclaims any liability, loss, injury, or damage incurred as a consequence, directly or indirectly, of the use and application of any of the contents of this text. Current Clinical Strategies is a registered trademark of Current Clinical Strategies Publishing Inc.

Current Clinical Strategies Publishing Inc
27071 Cabot Road
Laguna Hills, California 92653
Phone: 800-331-8227
FAX: 800-965-9420
E-mail: info@ccspublishing.com

Printed in USA   ISBN 1-881528-87-1

Table of Contents

Clinical Care of the HIV-Infected Patient

Primary HIV Infection

Acute retroviral syndrome occurs at the time the infection is acquired in 60% to 80% of HIV-infected persons. The illness resembles infectious mononucleosis from infection with Epstein-Barr virus (EBV), and acute retroviral syndrome is a consideration in differential diagnosis of heterophil-negative mononucleosis. Risk factors for transmission of HIV include history of a sexually transmitted disease, especially genital ulcers; unprotected anal or genital intercourse; and multiple sexual partners.

I. **Clinical signs and symptoms**
   A. The period between acquisition of HIV and onset of symptoms is about 14 days, and the characteristic signs and symptoms range from a mild fever and sore throat to a severe mononucleosis-type syndrome with high spiking fevers and a measles-like rash.
   B. In those patients with symptomatic seroconversion, the five most common signs and symptoms are fever, fatigue, pharyngitis, weight loss, and myalgias. Characteristic symptoms of acute retroviral syndrome occur in 50% to 90% of patients.

Differential Diagnosis of Primary HIV Infection

Epstein-Barr virus mononucleosis
Primary cytomegalovirus infection
Primary herpes simplex virus infection
Viral hepatitis
Rubella
Toxoplasmosis
Secondary syphilis
Measles
Disseminated gonococcal infection
Drug reaction

Signs and Symptoms of Primary HIV Infection	
Feature	**Frequency (%)**
Fever	95
Fatigue	90
Pharyngitis	70
Weight loss	68
Myalgias	60
Headache	58
Nausea	58
Cervical adenopathy	55
Night sweats	50
Diarrhea	50
Vomiting	40
Rash	35

II. Laboratory features

A. Primary HIV infection is diagnosed by a positive plasma HIV RNA obtained on the same day as a negative Western blot assay. If the interval between onset of symptoms and ordering of the HIV RNA test and Western blot assay is prolonged, both tests will be positive, suggesting that the patient has been infected with HIV for an extended period.

B. Clinical evaluation of possible primary HIV infection often includes a heterophil antibody (Monospot) test to rule out EBV mononucleosis, cytomegalovirus antigen or antibody, acute and convalescent serologic tests for rubella and toxoplasmosis, rapid plasma reagin test, Western blot assay for herpes simplex virus, and serologic tests for hepatitis (including hepatitis C virus RNA polymerase chain reaction). Because up to 30% of mononucleosis syndromes caused by EBV are heterophil-negative, other serologic tests for EBV may be necessary as well (eg, EBV IgM, IgG, early antigen, and nuclear antigens).

III. Initial management

A. When the diagnosis of primary HIV has been established, the patient should be examined for syphilis, herpes simplex, venereal warts, gonorrhea, and hepatitis.

B. If the patient is not infected with hepatitis A or B, vaccination should be considered. If the patient was identified as HIV RNA-positive and HIV EIA-negative, a follow-up HIV antibody test should be obtained 2 to 3 weeks after resolution of symptoms to establish that seroconversion has taken place.

C. A baseline CD4+ T-lymphocyte count should be obtained at the time of diagnosis. In the earliest stages of infection, the CD4+ count can sometimes be below 200 cells/µL. After the first several weeks of infection, a rebound in the CD4+ count to near normal levels may occur.

D. Baseline quantitative HIV RNA measurement should be obtained. In patients with severe symptoms of HIV seroconversion, viral titers may exceed 50 million copies/mL of blood. Viral titer falls rapidly after the first few weeks of infection, sometimes to undetectable levels.

IV. Therapy
   A. Therapy during primary HIV infection
   1. Viral loads are very high in the first weeks and months of HIV infection, and intervention at this time may ultimately result in a significant decrease in overall viral burden.
   2. The therapeutic regimen for acute HIV infection should include a combination of two nucleoside reverse transcriptase inhibitors and one potent protease inhibitor. Potential combinations of agents are much the same as those used in established infection and include the following regimens:
      a. Two nucleosides reverse transcriptase inhibitors plus a protease inhibitor2 NRTIs and 1 protease inhibitor
         (1) Zidovudine (AZT, Retrovir 300 mg PO bid) + lamivudine (3TC, Epivir 150 mg bid), didanosine (ddl, Videx), or zalcitabine (ddC, Hivid) + potent protease inhibitor (indinavir, Crixivan 800 mg q8h) or
         (2) Stavudine (d4T, Zerit) + lamivudine or didanosine + potent protease inhibitor
      b. Two nucleosides plus a non-nucleoside reverse transcriptase inhibitor:
         (1) Zidovudine (AZT, Retrovir) + lamivudine, didanosine, or zalcitabine + nevirapine (Viramune) or delavirdine mesylate (Rescriptor) or
         (2) Stavudine + lamivudine or didanosine + nevirapine or delavirdine.
   3. Triple-drug therapy may result in a significant clinical benefit when instituted as soon as possible after HIV acquisition. Once therapy is initiated it should be continued indefinitely because viremia may reappear or increase after discontinuation of therapy.
   B. Postexposure prophylaxis
   1. Combination chemotherapy results in fewer transmissions, and use of combination chemotherapy, including a protease inhibitor, is suggested following a significant intravenous exposure.
   2. Postexposure prophylaxis should also be initiated following sexual exposure.
   3. Postexposure prophylaxis treatment regimens
      a. Zidovudine (ZDV): 300 mg PO bid and
      b. Lamivudine (3TC, Epivir): 150 mg bid
      c. Protease Inhibitor: Indinavir (Crixivan) 800 mg q8h or Nelfinavir 750 mg tid (if needed to ensure 2 new antiviral drugs or for very risky exposure). §

References: See page 81.

Primary Care of HIV-Infected Adults

I. **Initial evaluation**
   A. The initial evaluation of the HIV-infected adult should include an assessment of the patient's past medical history, current symptoms and treatments, a complete physical examination, and laboratory testing.
   B. **Previous conditions**
      1. Prior medical conditions related to HIV infection should be assessed. Mucocutaneous candidiasis, oral hairy leukoplakia, hepatitis, pneumonia, sexually transmitted diseases, and tuberculosis should be sought. Past episodes of varicella-zoster, herpes simplex virus lesions, and opportunistic infections should be assessed.
      2. Dates and results of earlier tuberculin skin tests should be obtained. Women should be are asked about dates and results of Pap smears. Previous immunizations and antiretroviral therapy should be documented.
   C. **Current conditions and symptoms.** Fever, night sweats, unexplained weight loss, lymphadenopathy, oral discomfort, visual changes, unusual headaches, swallowing difficulties, diarrhea, dermatologic conditions, and respiratory and neurologic symptoms are suggestive of opportunistic infections or a malignant process.
   D. **Social history** includes information on past and present drug use, sexual behavior, dietary habits, household pets, employment, and current living situation. Residence and travel history should be assessed because coccidioidomycosis and histoplasmosis are more common in certain geographic regions.
II. **Physical examination**
   A. Weight, temperature, skin, oropharynx, fundi, lymph nodes, lungs, abdominal organs, genitalia, rectum, and the nervous system should be assessed. A cervical Pap smear should be obtained from women who have not had a normal result in the past year.
   B. Screening for Neisseria gonorrhoeae and chlamydial infection should be considered for sexually active men and women.
III. **Laboratory tests**
   A. **Complete blood count, chemistry profile, and serologic studies** for syphilis (rapid plasma reagin or VDRL), Toxoplasma gondii (IgG antibody), and hepatitis B (surface antigen, core antibody) should be obtained.
   B. Patients should have a tuberculin skin test unless they have been reactive in the past or have been treated for the disease. In HIV-infected persons, a positive test is 5 mm or more of induration.
   C. **A baseline chest film** is useful because many opportunistic pulmonary infections present with very subtle radiographic findings. A chest radiograph may suggest unrecognized tuberculosis.
   D. **CD4+ counts** assist in determination of the degree of immunologic damage, assess risk of opportunistic complications, and guide the use of prophylaxis against infections.
   E. **HIV RNA levels**
      1. Quantitation of plasma HIV RNA (viral load), a marker of the rate of viral replication, is useful in determining prognosis. It is used to estimate the risk of disease progression and to aid in making antiretroviral therapy decisions.

2. HIV RNA levels generally vary no more than 0.3 log in clinically stable patients. Sustained changes greater than threefold (0.5 log) are significant. A decrease occurs with successful antiretroviral therapy. A upward trend in a patient not receiving antiretroviral therapy indicates an increase in viral replication. Increases noted during treatment suggest antiretroviral drug failure or poor adherence.

Treatment Goals for HIV RNA Levels	
Parameter	**Recommendation**
Target level of HIV RNA after initiation of treatment	Undetectable; <5,000 copies/mL
Minimal decrease in HIV RNA indicative of antiretroviral activity	>0.5 log decrease
Change in HIV RNA that suggests drug treatment failure	Rise in HIV RNA level Failure to achieve desired reduction in HIV RNA level
Suggested frequency of HIV RNA measurement	At baseline: 2 measurements, 2-4 wk apart. 3-4 wk after initiating or changing therapy Every 3-4 mo in conjunction with CD4+ counts

3. HIV RNA levels should be obtained before the initiation or change of antiretroviral therapy. The next determination should be done a month after therapeutic intervention to assess its effect and then every 3 or 4 months.
4. Quantitative HIV RNA assays include branched DNA (bDNA) (Multiplex) and reverse transcriptase-initiated polymerase chain reaction (RT-PCR) (Amplicor HIV-1 Monitor). While both tests provide similar information, concentrations of HIV RNA obtained with the RT-PCR test are about twofold higher than those obtained by the bDNA method. For this reason, all HIV RNA determinations in a single patient should be obtained using the same assay.

IV. Prevention of infections
A. Vaccinations
1. Vaccination with pneumococcal vaccine, polyvalent (Pneumovax 23, Pnu-Immune 23) is recommended when HIV infection is diagnosed. Yearly influenza vaccination is suggested. Those who are seronegative for hepatitis B and at risk for infection should be offered hepatitis B vaccine (Recombivax HB, Engerix-B).
2. Tetanus vaccine should be administered every 10 years, and hepatitis A vaccine (Havrix, Vaqta) should be considered for nonimmune sexually active patients.

B. Opportunistic infections

1. **Pneumocystis carinii pneumonia** is rarely encountered in patients receiving prophylactic therapy. Indications for prophylaxis are a CD4+ count below 200 cells/μL, HIV-related thrush, or unexplained fever for 2 or more weeks regardless of CD4+ count. Anyone with a past history of PCP should continue suppressive therapy indefinitely because of the high risk of relapse.

2. **Toxoplasmosis** risk increases as the CD4+ count approaches 100 cells/μL, and patients who are seropositive for IgG antibody to toxoplasma should begin preventive therapy when the count nears this level. Patients who have been treated for toxoplasmosis require lifelong suppressive therapy.

USPHS/IDSA Guidelines for Prevention of Opportunistic Infections in HIV-Infected Patients

Pathogen	Indication for prophylaxis	First-choice drug	Selected alternative drugs
Prophylaxis Strongly Recommended			
Pneumocystis carinii	CD4+ count <200 cells/μL or unexplained fever for >2 wk or oropharyngeal candidiasis	TMP-SMX (Bactrim, Septra), 1 DS tablet PO daily	Dapsone, 100 mg PO daily, or aerosolized pentamidine (NebuPent), 300 mg monthly
Mycobacterium tuberculosis	Tuberculin skin test reaction of >5 mm or prior positive test without treatment or exposure to active tuberculosis	Isoniazid, 300 mg PO, plus pyridoxine, 50 mg PO daily for 12 mo	Rifampin, 600 mg PO daily for 12 mo
Toxoplasma gondii	IgG antibody to T gondii and CD4+ count <100 cells/μL	TMP-SMX, 1 DS tablet PO daily	Dapsone, 50 mg PO daily, plus pyrimethamine (Daraprim), 50 mg PO weekly, plus leucovorin (Welcovorin), 25 mg PO weekly
Mycobacterium avium complex	CD4+ <50 cells/μL	Clarithromycin (Biaxin), 500 mg PO bid, or azithromycin (Zithromax), 1,200 mg PO weekly	Rifabutin (Mycobutin), 300 mg PO daily
Streptococcus pneumoniae	All patients	Pneumococcal vaccine (Pneumovax 23, Pnu-Immune 23), 0.5 mL IM once	None

Consideration of Prophylaxis Recommended			
Hepatitis B virus	All seronegative patients	Hepatitis B vaccine (Engerix-B, 20 pg IM x 3, or Recombivax HB, 10 μg IM x 3)	None
Influenza virus	All patients, annually before influenza season	C.5 mL IM	Rimantadine (Flumadine), 100 mg PO bid, or amantadine (Symadine, Symmetrel), 100 mg PO bid

C. Tuberculosis. Patients who have HIV infection and positive results on tuberculin skin tests have a 2-10% per year risk of reactivation. If active tuberculosis has been excluded, prophylaxis should be prescribed to HIV-infected patients who have a tuberculin skin test reaction of 5 mm or more, who have a history of a positive tuberculin skin test reaction but were never treated, or who have had close contact with someone with active tuberculosis.

D. Mycobacterium avium complex infection. Prophylactic therapy is recommended for patients whose CD4+ counts are less than 50 cells/μL. Azithromycin (Zithromax), 1,200 mg (2 tabs) weekly by mouth is recommended.

E. Antiretroviral therapy
1. Antiretroviral drug regimens may suppress HIV replication almost completely in some patients. These changes are associated with improved survival and a lengthening in the time to development of AIDS-defining conditions.
2. HIV RNA levels are used to identify those patients who are at greatest risk for progression of disease and likely to benefit from antiretroviral therapy. HIV RNA quantitation also documents treatment efficacy and failure.

Antiretroviral Therapy

Initiate therapy for patients with:
Symptomatic HIV disease
Asymptomatic HIV disease but CD4+ count <500 cells/μL
HIV RNA levels >5,000 to 10,000 copies/mL

Consider therapy for patients with:
Detectable HIV RNA levels who request it and are committed to lifelong adherence

Recommended initial regimens:
2 NRTIs and 1 protease inhibitor
Zidovudine (AZT, Retrovir) + lamivudine (3TC, Epivir), didanosine (ddl, Videx), or zalcitabine (ddC, Hivid) + potent protease inhibitor or
Stavudine (d4T, Zerit) + lamivudine or didanosine + potent protease inhibitor
2 NRTIs and 1 NNRTI
Zidovudine (AZT, Retrovir) + lamivudine, didanosine, or zalcitabine + nevirapine (Viramune) or delavirdine mesylate (Rescriptor) or
Stavudine + lamivudine or didanosine + nevirapine or delavirdine

Change therapy for:
Treatment failure, as indicated by
Rising HIV RNA level
Failure to achieve target decrease in HIV RNA
Declining CD4+ count
Clinical progression
Toxicity, intolerance, or nonadherance

§

References: See page 81.

Antiretroviral Therapy

Antiretroviral treatment should be offered to all patients with the acute HIV syndrome, those within six months of seroconversion, and all patients with symptoms ascribed to HIV infection. In asymptomatic patients, treatment should be offered to individuals with fewer than 300 CD4[+] T cells/mm^3 or plasma HIV RNA levels exceeding 10,000 copies/mL (bDNA assay) or 20,000 copies/mL (RT-PCR assay). This may be achieved with a potent protease inhibitor (PI) in combination with two nucleoside analogue reverse transcriptase inhibitors (NRTIs).

I. **Plasma HIV RNA levels and CD4[+] T cell count**
   A. Measurement of plasma HIV RNA levels (viral load) should be performed at the time of diagnosis and every 3–4 months thereafter. Plasma HIV RNA levels should also be measured immediately prior to and at 2–8 weeks after initiation of antiretroviral therapy. A regimen of antiretroviral agents should result in a large decrease (~0.5 to 0.75 log$_{10}$) in viral load by 2–8 weeks.
   B. Once the patient is on therapy, HIV RNA testing should be repeated every 3–4 months. With optimal therapy viral levels in plasma should be undetectable (below 500 copies of HIV RNA per mL of plasma) at 6 months. If HIV RNA remains detectable after 6 months of therapy, the plasma HIV RNA test should be repeated to confirm the result, and a change in therapy should be considered. Plasma HIV RNA levels should not be measured during or within four weeks after treatment of any intercurrent infection, resolution of symptomatic illness, or immunization.

II. **Initiating therapy in asymptomatic HIV infection**
   A. Any patient with less than 500 CD4[+] T cells/mm^3 or greater than 10,000 (bDNA) or 20,000 (RT-PCR) copies of HIV RNA/mL of plasma should be offered therapy.

Indications for the initiation of antiretroviral therapy in the chronically HIV-infected patient		
Clinical Category	**CD4+ T Cell Count and HIV RNA**	**Recommendation**
Symptomatic (AIDS, thrush, unexplained fever)	Any value	Treat
Asymptomatic	CD4+ T Cells <500/mm^3 **or** HIV RNA >10,000 (bDNA) or >20,000 (RT-PCR)	Treatment should be offered.
Asymptomatic	CD4+ T Cells >500/mm^3 **and** HIV RNA <10,000 (bDNA) or <20,000 (RT-PCR)	Delay therapy and observe or treat.

Antiretroviral agents for treatment of HIV infection	
Column A	**Column B**
Indinavir	ZDV + ddI
Nelfinavir	d4T + ddI
Ritonavir	ZDV + ddC
Saquinavir	ZDV + 3TC
Ritonavir + Saquinavir	d4T + 3TC
Efavirenz	
Regimen should consist of agents from column A and column B	

III. Initiating therapy in advanced HIV disease. All patients diagnosed with advanced HIV disease (defined as any AIDS-defining condition) should be treated with antiretroviral agents. All patients with symptomatic HIV infection without AIDS, defined as the presence of thrush or unexplained fever, should also be treated. Once therapy is initiated, a maximally suppressive regimen, such as 2 NRTIs and a protease inhibitor, should be used.

IV. Indications for changing therapy
   A. Less than a 0.5–0.75 log reduction in plasma HIV RNA by 4 weeks following initiation of therapy, or less than a 1 log reduction by 8 weeks;
   B. Failure to suppress plasma HIV RNA to undetectable levels within 4–6 months of initiating therapy.
   C. Repeated detection of virus in plasma after initial suppression to undetectable levels.
   D. Any reproducible significant increase, defined as 3-fold or greater, from the nadir of plasma HIV RNA not attributable to intercurrent infection, vaccination, or test methodology;
   E. Persistently declining CD4$^+$ T cell numbers, as measured on at least two separate occasions; and
   F. Clinical deterioration. A new AIDS-defining diagnosis that was acquired after the time treatment was initiated suggests clinical deterioration.

Characteristics of nucleoside reverse transcriptase inhibitors (NRTIs)

Name	Zidovudine (*Retrovir*, AZT, ZDV)	Didanosine (*Videx*, ddI)	Zalcitabine (*HIVID*, ddC)	Stavudine (*Zerit*, d4T)	Lamivudine (*Epivir*, 3TC)
Dosage	200 mg tid or 300 mg bid or with 3TC as Combivir, 1 bid	>60kg: 200 mg bid <60 kg: 125 mg bid	0.75 mg tid	>60 kg: 40 mg bid < 60 kg: 30 mg bid	150 mg bid <50kg:2mg/kg bid or with ZDV as Combivir 1 bid
Adverse Events	Bone marrow suppression: Anemia and/or neutropenia, GI intolerance, headache, insomnia, asthenia Lactic acidosis with hepatic steatosis rare.	Pancreatitis, peripheral neuropathy nausea, diarrhea Lactic acidosis with hepatic steatosis rare.	Peripheral neuropathy, stomatitis Lactic acidosis with hepatic steatosis rare.	Peripheral neuropathy Lactic acidosis with hepatic steatosis rare.	Lactic acidosis with hepatic steatosis rare.

Characteristics of protease inhibitors

Name	Indinavir (*Crixivan*)	Ritonavir (*Norvir*)	Saquinavir (*Fortovase*)	Nolfinavir (*Viracept*)
Form	200, 400 mg caps	100 mg caps 600 mg/7.5ml po solution	200 mg caps	250 mg tablets 50mg/g oral powder
Dosage	800 mg q8h Take 1 hr before or 2 hrs after meals; may take with skim milk or low fat meal	600 mg q12h Take with food if possible	1,200 mg TID Take with food	750 mg TID Take with food

Name	Indinavir (Crixivan)	Ritonavir (Norvir)	Saquinavir (Fortovase)	Nelfinavir (Viracept)
Adverse Effects	Nephrolithiasis, GI intolerance, nausea, increased indirect bilirubinemia Headache, asthenia, blurred vision, dizziness, rash, metallic taste, thrombocytopenia, hyperglycemia, fat redistribution and lipid abnormalities	GI intolerance, nausea, vomiting, diarrhea Paresthesias - circumoral and extremities Hepatitis, asthenia, triglycerides increase >200%, transaminase elevation, elevated CPK and uric acid; hyperglycemia, fat redistribution and lipid abnormalities	GI intolerance, nausea, diarrhea, abdominal pain and dyspepsia Headache, elevated transaminase enzymes, hyperglycemia Fat redistribution and lipid abnormalities	Diarrhea, hyperglycemia Fat redistribution and lipid abnormalities
Drug Interactions	Inhibits cytochrome P450 Not recommended for concurrent use: rifampin, astemizole, cisapride, triazolam, midazolam, ergot alkaloids Levels increased by: ketoconazole, delavirdine, nelfinavir Levels reduced by: rifampin, rifabutin, grapefruit juice, nevirapine Didanosine: reduces indinavir absorption unless taken >2 hrs apart	Inhibits cytochrome P450 Increases levels of amiodarone, astemizole, bepridil, bupropion, cisapride, clorazepate, clozapine, diazepam, encainide, estazolam, flecainide, flurazepam, meperidine, midazolam, piroxicam, propoxyphene, propafenone, quinidine, rifabutin, triazolam, zolpidem, ergot alkaloids. Didanosine may cause reduced absorption; take >2 hours apart Decreases levels of ethinyl estradiol, theophylline, ZDV Increases levels of clarithromycin, desipramine	Inhibits cytochrome P450 Levels increased by: ritonavir, ketoconazole, grapefruit juice, nelfinavir, delavirdine Levels reduced by rifampin, rifabutin, phenobarbital, phenytoin, dexamethasone and carbamazepine, nevirapine Not recommended for concurrent use: rifampin, rifabutin, astemizole, cisapride, ergot alkaloids, triazolam, midazolam	Inhibits cytochrome P450 Levels reduced by rifampin, rifabutin Contraindicated: triazolam, midazolam, ergot alkaloids, astemizole, cisapride Nelfinavir decreases levels of ethinyl estradiol and norethindrone Nelfinavir increases levels of rifabutin, saquinavir and indinavir Not recommended for concurrent use: rifampin

Non-nucleoside reverse transcriptase inhibitors (NNRTIs)

Name	Nevirapine *(Viramune)*	Delavirdine *(Rescriptor)*	Efavirenz *(Sustiva)*
Form	200 mg tabs	100 mg tabs	50, 100, 200 mg capsules
Dosage	200 mg po qd x 14 days, then 200 mg po bid	400 mg po tid (four 100 mg tablets in >3 oz. water to produce slurry)	600 mg po qHS
Drug interactions	Induces cytochrome p450 enzymes The following drugs have suspected interactions that require careful monitoring if co-administered with nevirapine: rifampin, rifabutin, oral contraceptives, protease inhibitors, triazolam and midazolam	Inhibits cytochrome p450 enzymes Not recommended for concurrent use: astemizole, alprazolam, midazolam, cisapride, rifabutin, rifampin, triazolam, ergot derivatives, amphetamines, nifedipine, anticonvulsants (phenytoin, carbamazepine, phenobarbital) Delavirdine increases levels of clarithromycin, dapsone, quinidine, warfarin, indinavir, saquinavir Antacids or didanosine: separato delavirdine administration by >1 hr	Mixed inducer/inhibitor of cytochrome p450 A4 enzymes. Contraindications: astemizole, midazolam, triazolam, cisapride, ergot alkaloids. Efavirenz decreases indinavir, saquinavir, and increases levels of nelfinavir, ritonavir Potentially significant interactions: warfarin, clarithromycin, rifabutin, rifampin, ethinyl estradiol. Enzyme inducers such as rifampin, rifabutin, phenobarbital, and phenytoin decrease efavirenz concentrations.
Adverse Events	Rash Increased transaminase levels Hepatitis	Rash Headaches	Rash Central nervous systems symptoms Increased transaminase levels False positive cannabinoid test Teratogenic in monkeys

Drugs Available Through Treatment Investigational New Drug Protocols		
Drug	**Adefovir (Preveon)**	**Abacavir (1592-U89)**	**Amprenavir (Agenerase; 141W94)**
Class	Nucleotide RT Inhibitor	Nucleotide RT Inhibitor	Protease Inhibitor
Usual Dose	60 mg po qd or 120 mg po qd + L-carnitine 500 mg po qd	300 mg po bid	1200 mg po bid
Comments	Activity vs. HBV, CMV, HSV	Good CNS penetration; non CY450-mediated metabolism	Unique resistance profile

V. Therapeutic options when changing antiretroviral therapy

    A. A change in regimen because of treatment failure should involve complete replacement of the regimen with different drugs to which the patient is naive and to which cross-resistance is not anticipated. The new regimen may include the use of 2 new NRTIs and one new PI or NNRTI, two PIs with one or two new NRTIs, or a PI combined with an NNRTI.

Possible Regimens For Patients Who Have Failed Antiretroviral Therapy	
Prior Regimen	**New Regimen**
2 NRTIs +	2 new NRTIs
Nelfinavir (NFV)	RTV; or IDV; or SQV + RTV; or NNRTI RTV; or NNRTI + IDV
Ritonavir (RTV)	SQV + RTV**; NFV + NNRTI; or NFV + SQV
Indinavir (IDV)	SQV + RTV; NFV + NNRTI; or NFV + SQV
Saquinavir (SQV)	RTV + SQV; or NNRTI + IDV
2 NRTIs + NNRTI	2 new NRTIs + a protease inhibitor

§

References: See page 81.

Respiratory Symptoms in HIV-Infected Patients

Respiratory symptoms in HIV-infected individuals increase in frequency as the CD4 cell count declines below 200 cells/μL. Cough occurs at a frequency of 27%, shortness of breath at 23%, and fever at 9%.

Spectrum of Respiratory Illnesses in HIV-Infected Patients

Bacterial Infections
- Streptococcus pneumoniae
- Haemophilus influenzae
- Gram-negative bacilli (Pseudomonas aeruginosa, Klebsiella pneumoniae)
- Staphylococcus aureus

Mycobacterial Infections
- Mycobacterium tuberculosis
- Mycobacterium kansasii
- Mycobacterium avium complex

Fungal Infections
- Pneumocystis carinii
- Cryptococcus neoformans
- Histoplasma capsulatum
- Coccidioides immitis
- Aspergillus
- Candida species

Viral Infections
- Cytomegalovirus
- Herpes simplex virus

Parasitic Infections
- Toxoplasma gondii
- Strongyloides stercoralis

Neoplasms
- Kaposi's sarcoma
- Non-Hodgkin's lymphoma
- Bronchogenic carcinoma

Upper Respiratory Illnesses
- Upper respiratory tract infection
- Sinusitis
- Pharyngitis

Lower Respiratory Tract Disorders
    Lymphocytic interstitial pneumonitis (LIP)
    Nonspecific interstitial pneumonitis (NIP)
    Acute bronchitis
    Obstructive lung disease
    Asthma
    Chronic bronchitis
    Bronchiectasis
    Emphysema
    Pulmonary vascular disease
    Illicit drug-induced lung disease
    Medication-induced lung disease
    Primary pulmonary hypertension
    Bronchiolitis obliterans organizing pneumonia (BOOP)

VI. Diagnosis

A. **As the CD4 cell count declines below 500 cells/μL,** episodes of bacterial pneumonia may be recurrent, and mycobacteria other than M. tuberculosis (e.g. M. kansasii) may occur.

B. **At a CD4 cell count below 200 cells/μL,** bacterial pneumonia is often accompanied by bacteremia and sepsis, and M. tuberculosis infection is often extrapulmonary or disseminated. Pneumocystis carinii pneumonia and pneumonia/pneumonitis due to Cryptococcus neoformans become significant considerations.

C. **Below 100 cells/μL,** bacterial pathogens, such as Staphylococcus aureus and Pseudomonas aeruginosa, and pulmonary involvement from Kaposi's sarcoma or Toxoplasma gondii are increasingly diagnosed.

D. **At CD4 cell count <50 cells/μL,** respiratory diseases caused by endemic fungi (Histoplasma capsulatum, Coccidioides immitis), Cytomegalovirus, M. avium complex, and nonendemic fungi (Aspergillus, Candida) may occur.

CD4 Cell Count Ranges for Selected HIV-Related and Non-HIV-Related Respiratory Illnesses

Any CD4 cell count
    Upper respiratory tract illness
    Upper respiratory tract infection
    Sinusitis
    Pharyngitis
    Acute bronchitis
    Obstructive airway disease
    Bacterial pneumonia
    Tuberculosis
    Non-Hodgkin's lymphoma
    Pulmonary embolus
    Bronchogenic carcinoma

CD4 cell count <500 cells/μL
  Bacterial pneumonia (recurrent)
  Pulmonary mycobacterial pneumonia (nontuberculous)

CD4 cell count <200 cells/μL
  Pneumocystis carinii pneumonia
  Cryptococcus neoformans pneumonia
  Bacterial pneumonia (associated with bacteremia/sepsis)
  Disseminated or extrapulmonary tuberculosis

CD4 cell count <100 cells/μL
  Pulmonary Kaposi's Sarcoma
  Bacterial pneumonia (Gram-negative bacilli and Staphylococcus
  aureus increased)
  Toxoplasma pneumonitis

CD4 cell count <50 cells/μL
  Disseminated Histoplasma capsulatum
  Disseminated Coccidioides immitis
  Cytomegalovirus pneumonitis
  Disseminated Mycobacterium avium complex
  Disseminated mycobacterium (nontuberculous)
  Aspergillus pneumonia
  Candida pneumonia

VII. Symptoms
  A. Pneumocystis carinii pneumonia and pneumonia due to bacterial pathogens (most commonly Streptococcus pneumoniae and Haemophilus influenzae) are the two most likely HIV-related syndromes producing significant respiratory symptoms and pneumonia.
  B. Pneumocystis carinii pneumonia characteristically presents with fever, shortness of breath, and a dry, nonproductive cough. When the cough is productive, it is productive of clear phlegm/sputum. Respiratory symptoms are usually subacute and have been present for weeks.
  C. Pneumonia due to S. pneumoniae or H. influenzae characteristically presents with fevers, shaking chills or rigors, shortness of breath, pleuritic chest pain, and a productive cough with purulent sputum. Symptoms are usually acute and have been present for 3 to 5 days.

VIII. Past medical history
  A. Injection drug users are at risk for developing bacterial pneumonia and tuberculosis. Kaposi's sarcoma is seen almost exclusively in men who engage in sex with other men. Injection drug use or other illicit drugs can cause a variety of non-HIV-related pulmonary diseases (eg, endocarditis-related septic emboli or pneumonitis, respiratory depression, pulmonary edema).
  B. Cigarette smokers are at an increased risk for bacterial bronchitis, bronchopneumonia, and chronic obstructive lung disease.
  C. Travel to or residence in a geographic region that is endemic for one of the endemic fungi (Histoplasma capsulatum, Coccidioides immitis) increases the risk of disease.
  D. Tuberculosis exposure is more common in Asia and Latin America. HIV-infected patients from a country with a high prevalence of TB and patients

who are homeless, unstably housed, or previously incarcerated are at higher risk of exposure to M. tuberculosis. Patients who report or have a positive (> 5 mm in HIV-infected persons) purified protein derivative are at increased risk for TB, as are injection drug users.

E. **History of Pneumocystis carinii pneumonia** increases the risk for recurrence of PCP, and secondary P. carinii prophylaxis should be given to these patients. HIV-infected patients with a history of cryptococcosis, coccidioidomycosis, or histoplasmosis are at high risk for relapse and should receive life-long maintenance therapy.

IX. **Physical examination**

A. HIV-infected patients with pneumonia may be febrile, tachycardic, and tachypneic. Hypotension suggests a fulminant disease process. Pulse oximetry often reveals a decreased oxygen saturation and provides an estimate of the severity of the disease. The presence of exercise-induced desaturation, hypoxia, and/or an increase in the alveolar-arterial oxygen gradient is sensitive for Pneumocystis carinii pneumonia.

B. Pulmonary findings are absent in 50% of patients with Pneumocystis carinii pneumonia. Patients with bacterial pneumonia often have focal lung findings. Sudden onset of pleuritic chest pain, shortness of breath and absent breath sounds suggest a pneumothorax.

X. **Laboratory tests**

A. **White blood cell count (WBC)** is frequently elevated relative to the patient's baseline value in persons with bacterial pneumonia. HIV-infected patients with neutropenia are at higher risk of bacterial and fungal (Aspergillus, Candida species) infections. Persons with Pneumocystis carinii pneumonia may have an elevated, normal, or decreased WBC.

B. **Serum lactate dehydrogenase (LDH)** may suggest Pneumocystis carinii pneumonia. The serum LDH is frequently elevated in 83% of patients with Pneumocystis carinii pneumonia. The serum LDH may be elevated in many pulmonary and nonpulmonary conditions (including bacterial pneumonia), and patients with Pneumocystis carinii pneumonia may have a normal LDH level.

C. **Arterial blood gas (ABG).** Hypoxemia, an increased alveolar-arterial oxygen difference, and a respiratory alkalosis indicate significant pulmonary disease.

Chest Radiographic Findings in HIV-Related Disorders

Diffuse or multifocal infiltrates
Pneumocystis carinii
Bacteria
Mycobacterium tuberculosis
Fungi
Kaposi's sarcoma
Non-Hodgkin's lymphoma
Cytomegalovirus

Focal infiltrate
Bacteria
Mycobacterium tuberculosis
Fungi
Non-Hodgkin's lymphoma
Pneumocystis carinii

Reticular or granular pattern
Pneumocystis carinii
Cryptococcus neoformans
Bacteria (H. influenzae)
Other fungi (H. capsulatum)
Cytomegalovirus
Non-Hodgkin's lymphoma

Alveolar pattern
Bacteria
Mycobacterium tuberculosis (low CD4 cell count)
Cryptococcus neoformans
Non-Hodgkin's lymphoma
Pneumocystis carinii (uncommon unless severe, diffuse P. carinii)

Reticular or granular pattern
Pneumocystis carinii
Cryptococcus neoformans
Bacteria (H. influenzae)
Other fungi (H. capsulatum)
Cytomegalovirus
Non-Hodgkin's lymphoma

Miliary Pattern
Mycobacterium tuberculosis
Fungi (H. capsulatum, C. immitis, C. neoformans)
Pneumocystis carinii (uncommon)

Nodular pattern or nodule(s)
Mycobacterium tuberculosis
Fungi (C. neoformans, H. capsulatum, C. immitis, Aspergillus)
Kaposi's sarcoma (small nodules that gradually form larger,
coalescent nodules)
Non-Hodgkin's lymphoma (nodules/masses)
Bacteria
Pneumocystis carinii (less common)

Cyst(s)
Pneumocystis carinii
Fungi (especially C. neoformans and C. immitis)

Cavity(ies)
  Mycobacterium tuberculosis (usually high CD4 cell count)
  Bacteria (especially P. aeruginosa, S. aureus, R. equi)
  Fungi (Aspergillus species, C. neoformans, C. immitis)
  Mycobacterium kansasii
  Pneumocystis carinii (uncommon)

Pneumothorax
  Pneumocystis carinii
  Bacteria (uncommon)
  Mycobacterium tuberculosis (uncommon)

Intrathoracic adenopathy
  Mycobacterium tuberculosis
  Mycobacterium avium complex
  Fungi (C. neoformans, C. immitis, H. capsulatum)
  Kaposi's sarcoma
  Non-Hodgkin's lymphoma

Pleural effusion(s)
  Bacteria
  Mycobacterium tuberculosis
  Fungi (especially C. neoformans)
  Kaposi's sarcoma
  Non-Hodgkin's lymphoma

D. **Pneumocystis carinii pneumonia** presents with bilateral reticular or granular opacities. In mild cases, the radiograph may be normal. In patients with clinically suspected Pneumocystis carinii pneumonia who have a normal chest radiograph, high-resolution CT scan of the chest is a useful test. Patients with suspected Pneumocystis carinii pneumonia should undergo sputum induction and/or bronchoscopy to establish a definitive diagnosis.

E. **Bacterial pneumonia** due to Streptococcus pneumoniae characteristically presents in a bronchopneumonia pattern or with a focal segmental or lobar alveolar pattern, often with a pleural effusion.

F. **Tuberculosis** typically presents as upper lung zone infiltrates (apical and posterior segments of the upper lobes and superior segment of the lower lobes), often with cavities.

G. **Pulmonary Kaposi's sarcoma** presents with bilateral opacities in a central or perihilar distribution. §

References: See page 81.

Oral Complications of HIV Infection

Hairy leukoplakia is the most common oral lesion (20.4%) in HIV-infected patients. Candidiasis is the next most common lesion (5.8%).

I. **Candidiasis**
   A. Oral candidiasis (thrush) often precedes the development of AIDS in HIV-seropositive individuals. The most common form of oral candidiasis is pseudomembranous candidiasis, appearing as white plaques on any oral mucosal surface, which may be as small as 1 to 2 mm or may be widespread. Lesions can be wiped off, leaving an erythematous or bleeding mucosal surface.
   B. The erythematous form of candidiasis appears as smooth red patches on the hard or soft palate, buccal mucosa, or dorsal tongue. Angular cheilitis due to Candida infection produces erythema, cracks, and fissures at the corner of the mouth.
   C. Diagnosis of oral candidiasis is by potassium hydroxide preparation of a smear from the lesion.
   D. Oral candidiasis in patients with HIV infection usually responds to topical antifungal agents, including nystatin vaginal tablets (100,000 units tid, dissolved slowly in the mouth); nystatin oral pastilles (one 200,000 unit pastille five times daily).
   E. Ketoconazole (Nizoral), 200 mg PO once daily, is a systemic antifungal agent that can also be used. Fluconazole (Diflucan) is an extremely effective treatment for oral candidiasis, although resistance has been reported. Two 100-mg tablets are used on the first day, followed by one 100-mg tablet daily for 1 to 2 weeks.
   F. Angular cheilitis usually responds to topical nystatin-triamcinolone (Mycolog II), clotrimazole (Mycelex), or ketoconazole (Nizoral) cream.

Oral Lesions in HIV Infection	
Fungal Candidiasis Histoplasmosis Geotrichosis Cryptococcosis Aspergillosis	**Neoplastic** Kaposi's sarcoma Non-Hodgkin's lymphoma Squamous cell carcinoma
Bacterial HIV-associated gingivitis HIV-associated periodontitis Necrotizing stomatitis Mycobacterium avium complex Klebsiella stomatitis Bacillary angiomatosis	**Other** Recurrent aphthous ulcers Immune thrombocytopenic purpura Salivary gland disease

Viral Herpes simplex Herpes zoster Cytomegalovirus ulcers Hairy leukoplakia Warts	

II. Gingivitis and periodontitis

A. Gingivitis and periodontal disease is often seen in HIV infection, appearing as gingival erythema. Necrotizing ulcerative periodontitis occurs in 30% to 50% of AIDS patients.

B. Treatment involves débridement and curettage, followed by application of a topical antiseptic (povidone-iodine [Betadine]) irrigation, followed with chlorhexidine (Peridex) mouthwashes and a 4- to 5-day course of metronidazole (Flagyl) 250 mg qid or Augmentin 250 mg (1 tab tid).

III. Herpes simplex

A. Oral herpes lesions are a common feature of HIV infection, occurring as recurrent intraoral lesions with crops of small, painful vesicles that ulcerate. Lesions commonly appear on the palate or gingiva.

B. HSV can be identified using monoclonal antibodies and immunofluorescence. Treatment consists of oral acyclovir (one 200-mg capsule taken five times a day). Foscarnet is used for lesions that are resistant to acyclovir.

IV. Hairy leukoplakia

A. Hairy leukoplakia may affect the buccal mucosa, soft palate, and floor of mouth. It appears in all risk groups for AIDS, appearing as a white thickening of the oral mucosa, often with vertical folds or corrugations. The lesions range in size from a few millimeters to involvement of the entire dorsal surface of the tongue. Hairy leukoplakia is probably caused by a reactivation of Epstein-Barr virus.

B. The lesions will respond to high doses to acyclovir (Zovirax) 800 mg orally 5 times daily for 5 days. Valacyclovir (Valtrex) (1000 mg) or famciclovir (500 mg), given three times daily, is highly effective. For milder cases, topical applications of Retin-A or podophyllin may be helpful.

V. Kaposi's sarcoma

A. Kaposi's sarcoma may cause oral lesions in patients with AIDS, appearing as red or purple macules, papules, or nodules. Frequently they are asymptomatic; however, pain may result from traumatic ulceration, inflammation, or infection. Bulky lesions may interfere with speech and mastication. Diagnosis involves biopsy.

B. Treatment consists of surgical excision, local radiation, chemotherapy, or local injection of vinblastine.

VI. Recurrent aphthous ulcers

A. Recurrent aphthous ulcers are more common among HIV-positive individuals, appearing as recurrent crops of small (1-2 mm) to large (1-cm) ulcers on the oral and oropharyngeal mucosa.

B. Treatment consists of fluocinonide (Lidex), 0.05% ointment, mixed with equal parts of Orabase applied to the lesion up to six times daily, or clobetasol (Temovate), 0.05%, mixed with equal parts of Orabase applied three times daily.

C. Dexamethasone (Decadron) elixir, 0.5 mg/mL used as a rinse and expectorated, is also helpful. Thalidomide has been found to be useful in the management of steroid-resistant ulcers

References: See page 81.

Assessment of Fever in the HIV-Infected Patient

Infection is the most common cause of fever in AIDS patients. Diagnostic evaluation should first be directed at the possibility of infection or drug-induced fever.

I. **Clinical evaluation of fever in HIV-infected patients**
   A. Protracted unexplained fever is usually caused by either Pneumocystis carinii pneumonia, Mycobacterium avium complex, tuberculosis, sinusitis, cryptococcosis, or non-Hodgkin's lymphoma.
   B. In patients receiving prophylactic trimethoprim-sulfamethoxazole, P carinii pneumonia, toxoplasmic encephalitis, and salmonella bacteremia are less likely to occur.
   C. In patients with later-stage disease who develop significant and persistent fevers, MAC infection and lymphoma are common.
   D. Cryptococcal meningitis is a consideration in patients with fever accompanied by acute or chronic headache or changes in mental status.
   E. **Drug-induced fever**
      1. Drugs, such as penicillin derivatives, cephalosporins, Rifampin/Rifabutin, Dilantin, sulfa agents and drugs with sulfa side arms (eg, Lasix), INH, cimetidine, and tricyclic antidepressants.
      2. Drug-induced fever presents as high fever ($101°$) without proportionate tachycardia. The fever may be associated with rash, arthritis, or lymphadenopathy.
      3. The fever may occur even after long period of regular use of a drug and rarely may continue up to 2 weeks after offending agent is stopped.
      4. When there is no readily identifiable explanation for fever, discontinuation of recently initiated drugs should be attempted.
   F. **Primary HIV infection**
      1. Fever is the most common manifestation of symptomatic primary HIV infection. Additional findings include malaise, sweats, weight loss, arthralgia, myalgia, headache, pharyngitis, lymphadenopathy, and skin rash.
      2. The symptomatic primary infection resolves spontaneously, usually within 2 to 3 weeks.

II. **History**
   A. The patient's CD4 count is essential in assessing fever because different infections occur at different levels of immune function. Information from the patient's history may include residence in an area endemic for histoplasmosis or tuberculosis, or it may include failure to comply with anti-Pneumocystis prophylaxis.
   B. Men who do not engage in "safe sex" practices are predisposed to Salmonella bacteremia and to proctitis caused by herpes simplex virus, Treponema pallidum or Chlamydia trachomatis.
   C. Fever and inguinal adenopathy suggests infection caused by herpes simplex virus, C trachomatis, or T pallidum.

Causes of unexplained fever in HIV-infected patients

Any T cell range:
    Lymphoma
    Drug fever
    Extrapulmonary TB

T cells <200:
    Occult PCP
    Extrapulmonary pneumocystis
    Disseminated fungal disease

T cells <100:
    Mycobacterium avium complex
    Cytomegalovirus
    Visceral Kaposi's Sarcoma

III. Diagnostic approach to the febrile patient with a CD4+ count above 200 cells/μL

    A. Traditional bacterial infections (bronchitis, sinusitis, pneumonitis, bacteremia, pelvic inflammatory disease, pyelonephritis, cellulitis), viral respiratory infections, and tuberculosis (pulmonary, extrapulmonary) are the common causes of fever.

    B. P carinii pneumonia occasionally develops in HIV-infected patients with CD4+ counts above 200/μL; however, other opportunistic infections (cryptococcal meningitis, histoplasmosis, MAC, toxoplasma, cytomegalovirus) almost never occur at this stage.

    C. Laboratory evaluation of fever in HIV-infected patients

        1. Evaluation of fever includes a history and physical examination, a complete blood count, chest x-ray, urinalysis, blood cultures x 2, and liver enzyme tests (hepatitis), VDRL, and amylase.

        2. A tuberculin skin test should be done if PPD status is unknown.

        3. Blood cultures for fungi and mycobacterium (AFB) and a cryptococcal antigen test should be considered. Repeat cultures may be necessary to establish the diagnosis. Serum and urine testing for histoplasma antigen is also considered.

        4. Second tier studies: Gallium scan, abdominal CT scan, liver or bone marrow biopsy for diagnosis of MAI and disseminated fungal disease.

Diagnostic Studies for Fever in HIV-Infected Patients	
Cause	**Study**
Pneumocystis carinii pneumonia	Bronchoalveolar lavage

Disseminated Histoplasma capsulatum	Blood culture by lysis-centrifugation Bone marrow examination Antigen determination
Cryptococcal meningitis or disseminated disease	CSF, urine, blood cultures Blood, CSF antigen testing India ink preparation of CSF Tissue stains, cultures
Disseminated Toxoplasma gondii	Tissue stains PCR on blood samples Isolation of organism from CSF, blood, bronchoalveolar fluid
Disseminated mycobacterial disease	Blood culture Bone marrow examination, liver biopsy
Bartonella henselae	Blood or tissue culture

    D. If the patient is an injecting drug user, persistent fever may be caused by culture-negative endocarditis, osteomyelitis, or occult tuberculosis.

IV. HIV-infected patients with CD4+ counts below 200/μL

    A. Disorders noted above for less immunosuppressed patients should be considered plus neoplasms (non-Hodgkin's lymphoma) and opportunistic infections.

    B. Opportunistic infections include P carinii pneumonia or disseminated disease, disseminated infection with Histoplasma, cryptococcal meningitis or disseminated disease, Toxoplasma encephalitis or disseminated disease, disseminated mycobacterial (M avium complex, M genavense, M chelonei) disease, and Bartonella henselae infection.

    C. Investigation often reveals Pneumocystis carinii pneumonia, disseminated M avium complex, tuberculosis infection, or non-Hodgkin's lymphoma.

    D. Computed tomography is used for investigating central nervous system symptoms and for excluding sinusitis.

    E. Bone marrow aspiration for examination and culture is valuable for revealing opportunistic mycobacterial and fungal infections.

    F. Liver biopsy may provided a diagnosis of mycobacterial and cytomegalovirus infection in patients with unexplained fever and abnormal liver enzyme tests.

    G. Symptomatic management of fever. Sustained-release antipyretics, such as Indocin (75 mg PO bid) or Naprosyn (100 mg PO q daily) should be administered. Palliative prednisone may be considered in appropriate cases.

V. Specific pathogens causing fever

    A. Tuberculosis

        1. HIV patients who are injection drug users, immigrants, or who are close contacts of TB patients are predisposed to tuberculosis. HIV infection increases the risk of reactivating a latent infection.

        2. Although tuberculosis is primarily a pulmonary infection, HIV-infected patients with tuberculosis tend to demonstrate extrapulmonary disease.

3. Manifestations of pulmonary and extrapulmonary disease include fever, night sweats, weight loss, anorexia, chills, cough, headache, meningismus, hepatosplenomegaly, and lymphadenopathy.

4. To establish a diagnosis of tuberculosis, multiple sputum, stool, and urine specimens should be processed for acid-fast stains and cultures. In patients with advanced immunosuppression, M tuberculosis may sometimes be isolated from blood. Lumbar puncture, bone marrow aspiration, liver biopsy, and bronchoscopy may also be necessary.

5. Empirical antituberculous therapy can be prescribed while awaiting the results of smears and cultures.

B. **Mycobacterium avium complex infection**

1. MAC infections often manifest as persistent occult fever caused by disseminated infection. Clinical features include anorexia, weight loss, fever, night sweats, weakness, and diarrhea.

2. Risk for MAC begins at CD4 counts under $50/\mu L$. A fever without source in patients with such counts is most commonly due to MAC bacteremia.

3. Physical examination often will reveal hepatosplenomegaly along with cachexia. Laboratory abnormalities include anemia, leukopenia, and liver enzyme abnormalities.

4. The diagnosis can be established by mycobacterial blood culture. Two or three blood cultures drawn over a few days is sufficient.

5. The organism also can be cultured from of liver, bone marrow, or lymph node biopsy. The presence of MAC in stool or sputum is not diagnostic of invasive infection, but it should raise suspicion.

6. Patients with no other cause of fever and low CD4 counts may be started on a therapeutic/diagnostic trial looking for defervescence.

C. **Histoplasmosis**

1. This infection is a disseminated disease characterized by persistent fever and weight loss, often unassociated with respiratory symptoms.

2. The disease develops in patients who reside in endemic areas (Ohio, Mississippi River Valley, Indianapolis), or who have immigrated from endemic areas (Puerto Rico, Colombia, Dominican Republic), or who work in construction, or who have contact with caves, farms, or bird roost sites.

3. **Diagnostic studies** include serologic tests, isolation of the organism in body fluids and tissues, and recovery of the organism from blood, bone marrow, cerebrospinal fluid, or bronchoalveolar lavage fluid.

D. **Non-Hodgkin's lymphoma**

1. Systemic non-Hodgkin's lymphoma can cause fever accompanied by night sweats, fatigue, and weight loss. Systemic lymphomas usually develop at CD4+ counts less than $200/\mu L$.

2. Systemic lymphomas are characterized by widespread extranodal dissemination (to bone marrow, liver, meninges, GI tract) and by appearance at unusual sites (testes, parotid gland, gingiva, appendix).

3. Abnormalities that increase suspicion for non-Hodgkin's lymphoma include asymmetric or progressive lymphadenopathy, hepatomegaly, splenomegaly, unexplained GI symptoms, obstructive biliary disease, hilar adenopathy, an abdominal mass, elevated serum

alkaline phosphatase, markedly increased LDH level, or a sudden decrease in all peripheral blood cell lines.

References: See page 81.

Gastrointestinal Manifestations of HIV Disease

Gastrointestinal and hepatobiliary disorders are among the most frequent complaints in patients with HIV disease. Effective antiretroviral therapy and chemoprophylaxis (PCP, MAC, and CMV) has significantly reduced the occurrence of gastrointestinal opportunistic infections.

I. **Diarrhea**
   A. Diarrhea is the most common GI symptom in patients with HIV, affecting 0.9 to 14% of outpatients. Protozoal, viral, and bacterial organisms may cause diarrhea in patients with AIDS. MAC and CMV infections are observed in patients with CD4 cell count <100/mm^3. Pathogen-negative diarrhea is the cause of the most cases of diarrhea in this patient group.

Causes of Diarrhea in HIV-Infected Patients and Patients with Advanced HIV Disease

Protozoal/Helminth Infections
Cryptosporidium
Microsporidium
Isospora belli
Leishmania donovani
Giardia
Cyclospora
Entamoeba histolytica
Strongyloides stercoralis

Bacterial Infections
Mycobacterium avium complex
Salmonella
Shigella
Campylobacter sp.
Clostridium difficile
Small-bowel overgrowth
Vibrio parahaemolyticus

Viral Infections
Cytomegalovirus
Herpes simplex
Adenovirus
Picornavirus
HIV

Fungal Infections
Candida albicans
Histoplasma capsulatum

Neoplasms
Lymphoma
Kaposi's sarcoma

> **Idiopathic**
>   "AIDS enteropathy"

B. **Medications** are a common cause of diarrhea in patients with "early" HIV disease, especially protease inhibitors, such as nelfinavir and saquinavir. The diarrhea is often self-limited, lasting for 2 to 4 weeks from initiation of medication.

C. **Small Bowel Overgrowth**. Small bowel bacterial overgrowth may cause diarrhea and malabsorption of fat, vitamin B12, and carbohydrates. The prevalence of small bowel bacterial overgrowth with HIV-associated diarrhea is 38%.

D. **AIDS enteropathy**. HIV itself may be an indirect diarrheal pathogen. AIDS enteropathy causes diarrhea in HIV-infected patients who lack an identifiable pathogen.

E. **Evaluation of Diarrhea**

1. A careful history should exclude medications, lactose or food/fatty food intolerance, inadvertent use of cathartics (eg, megadoses of vitamin C, lactose-containing medications, sorbitol-containing foods), and symptoms suggestive of a systemic infection or neoplasm.

2. Cramps, bloating, and nausea suggest gastric or small-bowel involvement secondary to infection with Cryptosporidium, Microsporidium, Isospora belli, or Giardia. Hematochezia and tenesmus imply large-bowel inflammation resulting from CMV, Shigella, Campylobacter, or C. difficile infections. Tenesmus can occur as a result of herpes, Shigella, or Campylobacter infections.

3. Multiple sexual contacts or receptive anal intercourse increases the possibility of sexually transmitted diarrheal pathogens.

4. **Laboratory evaluation** should include stool culture for enteric bacteria, a specimen for Clostridium difficile toxin (in the setting of antibiotic use), and at least three stool specimens for ova and parasite examination (including acid-fast bacilli and trichrome stain). Three or more stool specimens should be tested. If a diagnosis is not reached following careful stool analysis, sigmoidoscopy is appropriate to identify CMV infection.

F. **Management of diarrhea in HIV disease**

1. Chronic administration of alternating antibiotics may be necessary for recurrent Salmonella, Shigella, Campylobacter, or Isospora infections. An empiric trial of oral antibiotics or antiparasite therapy for the possibility of small bowel overgrowth, undetected Campylobacter, Isospora enteritis, or undetected protozoa can be considered. Sulfonamides, ciprofloxacin, tetracyclines, or metronidazole may be effective.

Management of Diarrhea in HIV Disease			
Enteric Pathogen	**Clinical Features**	**Diagnosis**	**Treatment**
Mycobacter-ium avium complex	Blood culture, fever, severe anemia, night sweats, >10% weight loss, diarrhea, abdominal pain, hepatomegaly, increased alkaline phosphatase	Mycobacterial culture of blood and bone Mucosal biopsy	Rifabutin if CD4 <200 Azithromycin Clarithromycin Ethambutol Clofazimine Rifabutin Rifampin Ciprofloxacin
Cryptosporid-ium parvum	Non-bloody stool, diarrhea, nausea, vomiting, abdominal cramps	O and P	Paromomycin Spiramycin Erythromycin
Cytomegalo-virus	Submucosal hemorrhage, mucosal erosions, ulcerations, abdominal pain, diarrhea, bleeding, perforation, hematochezia	Mucosal biopsy	Ganciclovir Foscarnet
Microsporidia	Diarrhea	Mucosal biopsy	Albendazole

   2. Chronic diarrhea should be treated symptomatically with Imodium, Lomotil, or tincture of opium drops. Lactose-containing foods should be avoided as a diagnostic trial. Bulk-forming agents, including effersyllium, bran and pectin, may be helpful.
   3. Octreotide, a subcutaneous somatostatin analogue, is particularly effective in patients with diarrhea who lack a specific infection.

II. **Dysphagia and odynophagia**
   A. Dysphagia, odynophagia, or both, due to esophagitis are very common in advanced HIV disease. The majority of patients with dysphagia or odynophagia have candidal esophagitis. Malignancies, such as KS and lymphoma, and acid-reflux esophagitis can also occur.
   B. Candida and herpes esophagitis are predominantly identified in patients with CD4 cell counts less than 200 cells/nm^3. CMV and idiopathic ulcers are noted below a CD4 cell count of 100 cells/mm^3.
   C. **Evaluation of dysphagia and odynophagia**. Endoscopy with biopsy is the best method of establishing a specific etiology.
   D. **Treatment of dysphagia and odynophagia**
      1. Patients with odynophagia who have oral thrush should be treated empirically with fluconazole (Diflucan),100 to 200 mg/day or itraconazole (Sporanox), 200 mg/day.
      2. Refractory Candida esophagitis requires treatment with amphotericin B. Herpes esophagitis responds to acyclovir (200-mg capsules every 4 hours). Acyclovir-resistant herpes may respond to foscarnet. Infections with CMV generally respond to a 2- to 3-week course of ganciclovir.

3. Nonspecific ulcerations may be treated with a short course of oral corticosteroids (40 mg/day, tapered over 3 weeks) or thalidomide (200 mg/day), or with H-2 antagonists and sucralfate. §

References: See page 81.

Neurologic Manifestations of HIV Infection

Involvement of the nervous system in HIV infection is common, manifesting in about half of patients.

I. **Neurologic complications**
   A. **Aseptic meningitis.** At the time of HIV seroconversion or primary infection, patients may present with symptoms of aseptic meningitis, such as fever, headache, stiff neck, and a lymphocytic pleocytosis.
   B. **AIDS dementia complex**
      1. AIDS dementia complex is reported in about 6% to 7% of patients with AIDS. Clinical features include cognitive cysfunction, impaired motor performance, and behavioral changes. Subclinical cognitive and motor impairment may occur at all stages of HIV infection.
      2. Progressive symptoms may include mental slowing, forgetfulness, poor concentration, apathy, social withdrawal, loss of spontaneity, and reduced libido. Patients display personality changes, including reduced emotional expression, increased irritability, mania, and disinhibition. Loss of fine motor control (deterioration in handwriting), slowing of gait, unsteadiness, urinary incontinence, and tremor may be seen. Seizures occur in 10% of patients.
      3. AIDS dementia complex is a diagnosis of exclusion because depression, metabolic disorders, and other infectious causes of encephalitis may present in a similar manner. Clinical diagnosis may be aided by neuropsychologic testing.
      4. Central nervous system (CNS) computed tomography (CT) and magnetic resonance imaging (MRI) are used to exclude other treatable conditions. They may reveal cerebral atrophy.
      5. AIDS dementia complex may respond to highly active antiretroviral therapy, which should include of at least one agent that has significant CNS penetration.
   C. **Myelopathy**
      1. HIV-related spinal cord involvement is uncommon. It presents as spastic paraparesis with bowel and bladder dysfunction, gait ataxia, and variable sensory loss, usually in the context of advanced immunodeficiency.
      2. Diagnosis must exclude cord-compression lesions (eg, lymphoma, epidural abscess), vitamin B12 deficiency, and other viral infections (eg, human T-cell lymphotropic virus type I varicella-zoster virus, cytomegalovirus).
      3. Myelopathy may respond to highly active antiretroviral therapy. Additional treatment should be directed at ameliorating symptoms.
   D. **Distal symmetric polyneuropathy**
      1. Distal sensory polyneuropathy may develop as a consequence of HIV infection, but it is more commonly associated with use of antiretroviral agents, specifically zalcitabine (HIVID), didanosine (Videx), and stavudine (Zerit). It tends to occur with advanced infection. Symptoms typically consists of distal paresthesias, with burning sensations and numbness of fingertips and toes, that progress proximally.
      2. Physical examination reveals diminished ankle reflexes and decreased sensation to pinprick, light touch, and vibration. Nerve-conduction tests demonstrating axonal neuropathy can confirm the diagnosis. The possibility of vitamin B12 deficiency should be

      excluded.

   3. Management consists of dose reduction or discontinuation of any potentially offending agents. Symptomatic treatment with tricyclic antidepressants, anticonvulsants (eg, carbamazepine, gabapentin [Neurontin]), lidocaine 30% cream, and narcotic analgesics may be effective.

II. Infectious processes

A. Cerebral toxoplasmosis

   1. Cerebral toxoplasmosis occurs as a consequence of reactivation, developing in about 2% to 10% of patients with HIV infection and prior toxoplasma infection (identified by positive IgG titers). Most cases occur when the CD4+ T-lymphocyte count is less than 100 cells/μL.

   2. Clinical manifestations include headache, confusion, fever, focal neurologic deficits, and seizures. CT and MRI reveal lesions with ring enhancement. Lesions are often multiple with associated mass effect involving the frontal and parietal lobes and basal ganglia. Characteristic CT or MRI findings and positive serologic results are indications for empirical therapy. Definitive diagnosis is by brain biopsy.

   3. Treatment regimens consisting of sulfadiazine or of clindamycin (Cleocin) plus pyrimethamine (Daraprim) for 6 weeks have been equally effective. Clinical improvement is usually seen in 10 to 14 days. Lifetime suppressive therapy is recommended.

   4. Patients at risk for toxoplasmosis (CD4+ count less than 100 cells/μL and positive serology) should be offered primary prophylaxis with trimethoprim-sulfamethoxazole (Bactrim, Septra) or dapsone plus pyrimethamine.

B. Cryptococcal meningitis

   1. Cryptococcus neoformans can cause fungal meningitis in the presence of HIV infection, usually in patients with a CD4+ count less than 100 cells/μL. The organism disseminates widely, with predilection for the CNS.

   2. Headache and fever are the most common presenting symptoms; others include nausea and vomiting, photophobia, blurred vision, stiff neck, skin lesions, altered mentation, and seizures.

   3. CSF culture confirms the diagnosis. India ink preparations of CSF and cryptococcal antigen testing of serum and CSF are usually positive. Blood cultures are positive in only about one fourth of cases. Neuroimaging may reveal cryptococcomas, hydrocephalus, and cerebral edema. The mortality rate of cryptococcal meningitis is 10% to 20%.

   4. Antifungal treatment regimens include either amphotericin B (Fungizone) and flucytosine (Ancobon) or amphotericin B alone for 2 weeks, followed by daily fluconazole (Diflucan).

   5. Elevated intracranial pressure should be aggressively managed with CSF drainage by lumbar puncture, ventriculoperitoneal shunting, and acetazolamide (Diamox). Long-term suppression with fluconazole is recommended to avoid recurrence.

C. Progressive multifocal leukoencephalopathy

   1. Reactivation of latent JC virus results in progressive multifocal leukoencephalopathy. This condition usually occurs when CD4+ counts are less than 100 cells/μL. Clinical features are subacute in onset and include limb weakness, impairment of cognitive function,

      gait disturbance, incoordination, speech and visual disturbances, headache, and seizures.

2. CT typically shows hypodense white-matter lesions, usually parietooccipital, with no enhancement or mass effect. MRI may more clearly show lesions.

3. A positive CSF polymerase chain reaction for JC virus is diagnostic; however, a negative result cannot exclude the diagnosis. The prognosis of progressive multifocal leukoencephalopathy is poor. Remission with potent antiretroviral therapy may occur.

D. CMV encephalitis

1. In patients with a CD4+ T-lymphocyte count less than 100 cells/μL, CMV disease develops within 2 years in 21.4%. The usual presentation consists of retinitis and esophagitis, with or without colitis; pneumonitis, hepatitis, encephalitis, and polyradiculopathy also may occur.

2. Clinical features of encephalitis include rapidly progressive confusion, delirium, apathy, and focal neurologic deficits. CT may reveal diffuse low-attenuation areas. MRI reveals high signal intensity lesions on T2-weighted images. Periventricular enhancement and edema are characteristic. CSF yields nonspecific findings.

3. Polyradiculopathy manifests as lower extremity weakness, paresthesias, and bladder and bowel dysfunction. Saddle pain and urinary retention are common. Elevated protein level and polymorphonuclear pleocytosis are noted on CSF analysis. Detection of CMV DNA on CSF polymerase chain reaction testing is diagnostic.

4. Ganciclovir sodium (Cytovene) and foscarnet (Foscavir) have had variable effectiveness in treatment of CMV infection of the CNS.

E. Neurosyphilis

1. In patients with HIV infection, neurosyphilis develops within a shorter interval. The prevalence of syphilitic meningitis, uveitis, and hearing loss is increased.

2. Asymptomatic patients with positive serologic findings should undergo CSF examination for exclusion of neurosyphilis.

III. Neoplasm

A. Lymphoma in the CNS occurs in 5% of patients with AIDS, usually late in the disease course. Manifestations may include headaches, mental status changes, seizures, and focal neurologic signs and symptoms.

B. Lesions most commonly affect the periventricular gray and white matter; most are supratentorial, but some are multifocal. CT and MRI reveal single or multiple discrete mass lesions with diffuse homogeneous contrast enhancement and some mass effect.

C. Thallium 201 single-photon emission CT of the brain can help distinguish lymphoma from toxoplasmosis, but brain biopsy is required for diagnosis.

D. Prognosis of CNS lymphoma is poor. Response of lesions to radiation therapy is variable. §

References: See page 81.

Dermatologic Manifestations of HIV Infection

I. Infectious cutaneous conditions
  A. **Staphylococcus aureus infections**
    1. Staphylococcus aureus is the most common bacterial skin infection in persons with HIV disease.
    2. **Bullous impetigo**. Bullous impetigo is most common in hot, humid weather, presenting as very superficial blisters or erosions, most commonly seen in the groin or axilla.
    3. **Ecthyma** is an eroded or superficially ulcerated lesion with an adherent crust. Purulent material is present under this crust.
    4. **Folliculitis**
      a. Folliculitis due to S. aureus occurs most commonly in the hairy areas of the trunk, groin, axilla, or face. Gram's stain and culture of pustules confirms the diagnosis.
      b. Often the follicular lesions of the trunk are intensely pruritic and may be mistaken for scabies. About 50% of HIV-infected persons with scabies have coexistent S. aureus folliculitis.
    5. **Treatment of cutaneous staphylococcal lesions**
      a. Very superficial lesions, like bullous impetigo, often respond to an antistaphylococcal antibiotic, such as dicloxacillin (500 mg given PO qid) or 7-10 days. Combinations of antibiotics, especially a dicloxacillin or cephalexin (Keflex) plus rifampin (600 mg once daily), are often necessary.
      b. Washing the infected area once daily or every other day with an antibacterial agent (Hibiclens, Betadine) helps remove crusts, dries lesions, and decreases surface bacterial concentration. Topical antibiotics (clindamycin 1% or erythromycin 2% solutions) applied twice daily may be used.
      c. Loculated abscesses must be incised and drained when fluctuant. Intravenous antibiotics are required when significant cellulitis of or symptoms of bacteremia are present, appropriate. Intranasal mupirocin may reduce carriage rate and prevent relapses. Chronic oral antibiotics may be required to prevent relapse.
  B. **Bacillary angiomatosis**
    1. Bacillary angiomatosis is an infection caused by two species of Bartonella - B. henselae and B. quintana. These bacteria are extremely difficult to culture. One of the agents causing bacillary angiomatosis, B. henselae, is associated with cat scratch disease. Cat exposure and cat scratches are risk factors for acquiring bacillary angiomatosis.
    2. Visceral disease may include osseous lesions, hepatic and splenic involvement, lymph node disease, pulmonary lesions, brain lesions, and widespread fatal systemic involvement.
    3. **Clinical Features**
      a. Bacillary angiomatosis is characterized by pyogenic granulomas -- fleshy, friable, protuberant papules-to-nodules that tend to bleed very easily. In addition, deep cellulitic plaques and subcutaneous nodules may occur. Lesions number from a few to hundreds. Diagnosis is confirmed by biopsy.
      b. Fever, night sweats, weight loss, and anemia are common. Involvement of the liver and spleen is the most commonly

diagnosed form of visceral disease. These patients present with abdominal pain, fevers, elevated levels on liver function tests, and hepatosplenomegaly.
4. **Treatment.** Erythromycin (500 mg orally 4 times daily) or doxycycline (100 mg orally twice daily) is effective. Therapy should continue for 8 weeks. Patients with visceral disease should receive 4 months of therapy.

C. Herpes simplex virus
1. Chronic persistent infection with herpes simplex virus (HSV) is common in patients with advanced HIV disease and is a Centers for Disease Control (CDC)-defined index infection in establishing an AIDS diagnosis.
2. Lesions may appear as grouped blisters that rupture, crust, and heal in 7 to 10 days. Once severely immunosuppressed, HIV-infected persons often experience chronic lesions that continue to expand and form large, painful ulcers and crusted erosions, 2 to 10 cm or larger.
3. Periungual infection is another characteristic manifestation of HSV-2 infection in the HIV-infected patient; all paronychial lesions should be cultured for HSV.
4. Fluorescent antibody testing or viral culture of fresh lesions are diagnostic.
5. **Treatment**
   a. **Acyclovir** (Zovirax, 200 to 400 mg orally 5 times daily) should be prescribed until the ulcers heal, which may take several weeks. Chronic suppressive therapy may be instituted with acyclovir (400 mg orally twice daily) to reduce recurrences. Famciclovir (Famvir, 250 mg 3 times daily) and valacyclovir (Valtrex, 100 mg twice daily) have higher bioavailability and require less frequent dosing.
   b. **Acyclovir-Resistant HSV Infection.** Large chronic perianal, perioral, or periungual ulcers that fail to heal with acyclovir are often caused by acyclovir-resistant HSV-2. Treatment with foscarnet and continuous-infusion acyclovir is beneficial. Trifluridine ophthalmic solution may be effective for lesions that do not respond to acyclovir and foscarnet.

D. Varicella zoster infection
1. Varicella zoster virus (VZV) infection is commonly seen early in the course of HIV infection.
2. This dermatomal eruption may be particularly bullous, hemorrhagic, necrotic, and painful in HIV-infected persons. The duration of blisters and crusts is usually 2 or 3 weeks.
3. Dissemination of VZV in HIV infection is uncommon. The clinical manifestations of disseminated VZV infection include typical blisters with or without an associated dermatomal eruption.
4. **Treatment**
   a. **Oral acyclovir.** If the patient has a reasonably intact immune system and does not have clinical features of disseminated or visceral infection, and if lesions are not near the eye (trigeminal nerve), then oral acyclovir is adequate. A dosage of 800 mg orally 5 times daily for 5 days is recommended
   b. **Famciclovir (Famvir),** 500 mg, and **valacyclovir (Valtrex),** 1000 mg, may be given only three times daily but the dosage must be adjusted in renal impairment.
   c. **Intravenous acyclovir** (10 mg/kg 3 times daily) is indicated when

the immunosuppression is significant (CD4 <200), when disseminated or visceral lesions are present, and when VZV affects the ophthalmic branch of the trigeminal nerve (eyelid or tip of the nose). Intravenous treatment should continue until the lesions are well crusted (usually about 7 days), after which full doses of oral acyclovir may complete 10 to 14 days of therapy.

   d. Wet compresses (2 or 3 times daily) will help remove necrotic debris. Silver sulfadiazine (Silvadene) or bacitracin keeps the scabs soft and may also prevent secondary infection. Capsaicin cream (Zostrix) may reduce the pain of both acute and chronic zoster. It may be applied to the lesions 5 times daily until the pain is controlled.

E. Molluscum contagiosum

  1. Molluscum contagiosum is a superficial cutaneous viral infection manifesting as 2- to 3-mm flesh-colored hemispheric papules. A faint whitish core usually is visible at the center of each papule, some of which may be slightly umbilicated. This eruption is seen commonly in immunocompetent young children (ages 3 to 8 years), whose lesions are scattered widely over the face, arms, and trunk. In adults, this mild infection is usually sexually transmitted and occurs in the pubic area.

  2. Genital molluscum in the non-HIV-infected adult may be chronic, and it occurs in 10 to 20% of HIV-infected persons. Early in the infection, the lesions are usually mild and localized to the groin or face. Lesions tend to proliferate once CD4 counts fall below 200. They often number greater than 100 and may involve the face, trunk, and groin; there is a predilection for the eyelids.

  3. Treatment. Light cryotherapy using liquid nitrogen can treat individual lesions. If this is not available, pricking the lesion with a large-gauge needle and removing the white core may also be effective. For refractory lesions, removal by curettage without cautery is very effective.

F. Human papillomavirus (warts)

  1. Superficial cutaneous infection with human papillomavirus (HPV) occurs with increased frequency in immunosuppressed patients. The warts seldom cause symptoms, except when on the soles of the feet and around the fingernails.

  2. Relapse of warts after treatment is common, especially in advanced HIV disease. Liquid nitrogen cryotherapy can be applied every 2 to 4 weeks. Topical "anti-wart" medications containing salicylic and lactic acids are applied daily under occlusion and may lead to complete disappearance of the lesions. The treatment outlook for warts is poor in immunosuppressed patients.

  3. Topical treatment of genital warts with podophyllin or trichloroacetic acid may be applied weekly for 6 to 10 weeks. Liquid nitrogen freezing has a slightly greater response rate. Recurrence is almost universal.

  4. The presence of external genital warts in women and perirectal warts in homosexual or bisexual men is usually associated with internal warts. Pelvic examination, Pap smear, and colposcopy are recommended in women, and anoscopy in men.

G. Acute HIV exanthem and enanthem

  1. In acute primary HIV infection, a rash may develop along with a

mononucleosis-like illness. The rash may be exanthematous or pityriasis rosea-like, usually does not itch, is distributed over the upper trunk and proximal limbs, and may involve palms and soles. An associated enanthem of oral erythema or superficial erosions may be present. The exanthem and enanthem spontaneously resolve within 1 to 2 weeks.
   2. Detection of HIV antigen by enzyme immunoassay may confirm the diagnosis of acute HIV infection in HIV-antibody-negative persons.
H. **Syphilis**
   1. Cutaneous presentations of primary and secondary syphilis in HIV-infected persons are usually similar to those in non-HIV-infected persons. HIV may delay development of serologic evidence of Treponema pallidum, resulting in negative tests. In the HIV-infected person, a negative serologic test may not be adequate to rule out secondary syphilis.
   2. **Treatment**. HIV infected patients with early syphilis should be treated with weekly intramuscular injections of penicillin G benzathine (Bicillin) 2.4 million units for 2 or 3 weeks. CSF examination is required if there are any clinical findings suggesting CNS involvement.
   3. Quantitative nontreponemal tests are repeated at 1, 2, and 3 months and thereafter at 3-month intervals until a satisfactory serologic response occurs. If an appropriate fall in titer does not occur (two dilutions by 3 months for primary or by 6 months in secondary).
II. **Inflammatory skin conditions**
   A. **Eosinophilic folliculitis**
      1. Eosinophilic folliculitis typically occurs in HIV-infected persons with helper T cell counts below 200. Intensely pruritic, edematous, urticarial papules and pustules appear in crops on the trunk or face or both. Cultures and histologic examination for infectious agents are negative, but a relative peripheral eosinophilia may be present.
      2. Astemizole (Hismanal), 10 mg daily has been used with limited success, but concurrent imidazole or erythromycin therapy is contraindicated with astemizole because of the risk of cardiac arrhythmia. Ultraviolet phototherapy is also beneficial. Itraconazole in a dosage of 200 to 400 mg daily is sometimes beneficial. Permethrin 5% (Elimite) used every other day from the waist up may bring improvement in some patients: Permethrin kills the Demodex mite, which may be the etiologic agent in eosinophilic folliculitis.
   B. **Drug reactions**
      1. The incidence of adverse reactions TMP-SMX is very high. Most reactions occur in the second week of therapy, and the rash is a maculopapular/morbilliform reaction, beginning in the groin and pressure areas and quickly generalizing. Cutaneous eruptions occur in 48% of treated patients. Resolution of the skin rash during therapy occurs in 33%, and the remaining patients have progressive toxicity, necessitating discontinuation of the drug.
      2. The use of systemic corticosteroids in treating PCP reduces the rate of drug eruption from TMP-SMX. Other drug-induced hypersensitivity reactions include urticarial reactions, exfoliative erythroderma, fixed-drug eruption, erythema multiforme, and toxic epidermal necrolysis. These reactions are most often due to antibiotics, especially TMP-SMX and the penicillins.

C. Scabies

1. Scabies usually presents with pruritic papules with accentuation in the intertriginous areas, genitalia, and fingerwebs. Gamma-benzene hexachloride (lindane) applied from the neck down for 8 to 24 hours is usually curative; however, that lindane may result in peripheral neuropathies in HIV-infected patients, particularly in those with CD4 < 200. In patients with scabies who have not responded to gamma-benzene hexachloride therapy, 5% permethrin cream (Elimite), used in the same method as lindane, is safe and effective.

2. True crusted (Norwegian) scabies may occur in patients with advanced HIV disease. Norwegian scabies is nonpruritic and appears as thick crusts. The crusts are highly contagious. Treatment with Elimite should be repeated at least weekly until cutaneous manifestations clear. Ivermectin, 6% precipitated sulfur ointment, daily should be added to the Elimite therapy.

III. Kaposi's sarcoma

A. Kaposi's sarcoma is a neoplasm of endothelial cells within the skin and other organs. Most KS patients are homosexual men. KS may be present in up to 46% of homosexual men with advanced HIV disease at initial diagnosis. The incidence in heterosexual injection drug users is only 3.8%. Herpes virus 8 (HHV-8) has been associated with KS. Most individuals with KS have generalized, slowly progressive disease; others have stable KS.

B. KS may affect any portion of the cutaneous surface. Initially, it appears as red-to-brown flat macules. Papules, nodules, and tumors may also be present or develop later. Numbering from one to hundreds, they range in size from several millimeters to over 10 cm and may be widespread, grouped, or zosteriform. KS may affect mucosal surfaces and internal organs. Visceral involvement occurs in 72% of patients with advanced HIV disease and KS, most often affecting the gastrointestinal tract (50%), lymph nodes (50%), and lungs (37%).

C. Biopsy of the skin establishes the diagnosis. A 3.5- to 4.0-mm punch biopsy should be taken from the center of the lesion.

D. Treatment. If treatment is necessary, radiation and systemic alpha-interferon or chemotherapy may be used. Cutaneous lesions may improve with local cryotherapy or intralesional injections of vinblastine, 0.2 to 0.6 mg/mL.

References: See page 81.

Psychiatric Disorders in HIV-infected Patients

I. **Delirium**
   A. Delirium is the clinical manifestation of a CNS metabolic disturbance. Systemic illness, CNS infection or neoplasm, and medications may cause delirium in advanced HIV disease. Hypoxia, dehydration, sepsis, renal failure, hyponatremia, hypercalcemia, and hypoglycemia can cause delirium. Delirium may be caused by HIV encephalopathy, cryptococcal meningitis, neurosyphilis, progressive multifocal leukoencephalopathy, herpes encephalitis, cytomegalovirus encephalitis, disseminated toxoplasmosis, lymphoma, and trauma.
   B. **Medications associated with delirium.** Anticholinergics, antihistamines, sedatives, opioids and antibiotics (cephalosporins and amphotericin B, antineoplastics) can cause delirium. Delirium may be the result of intoxication or withdrawal from abused substances, including alcohol, stimulants, hallucinogens sedatives, and opiates.
   C. **Early symptoms** of delirium include irritability and sleep-wake cycle alterations. A later symptom of delirium is rapid onset of fluctuating level of consciousness, with markedly poor attention and disorganized thought and speech. Orientation and memory are often impaired. Illusions may be present. The patient may be agitated or apathetic.
   D. **Treatment of delirium**
      1. Treatment consists of treatment of the underlying disease process and identification of medications contributing to the confusional state.
      2. **Olanzapine (Zyprexa)**, an "atypical" neuroleptic with a very low incidence of extrapyramidal symptoms, is effective for treatment of agitation accompanying delirium. Treatment should start at 2.5 mg bid or 5 mg qhs, and increasing up to 20 mg po qhs as needed. Olanzapine can lower seizure thresholds, but otherwise is well tolerated.
      3. **Risperidone (Risperdal)** is also effective and well-tolerated, starting at 0.5 twice a day or 1 mg at bedtime, increasing up to 3 mg twice a day if necessary.
      4. **Haloperidol (Haldol)** may be used at low doses (0.5 to 2.0 mg 2 times a day) when intravenous administration is necessary. Extrapyramidal side effects are common. Additional sedation can be obtained with lorazepam (Ativan), starting at 0.5 to 1.0 mg every 3 to 8 hours as needed.
      5. **Nonpharmacologic treatments** include assisting with orientation by having a calendar and clock in the patient's room, and keeping the patient's room well lit when the patient is awake.

II. **Cognitive impairment and dementia**
   A. Neurocognitive impairment is common in persons with advanced HIV disease. Early symptoms include poor concentration, psychomotor slowing, difficulty with complex sequential motor activity, apathy, and withdrawal. Advanced dementia may manifest as severe cognitive deficits, disinhibition, mutism and/or catatonia, ataxia, and incontinence.
   B. **Treatment of dementia** consists of treatment of the underlying organic cause. Multidrug regimens to lower serum viral load, which include protease inhibitors, often will slow progression and may even reverse HIV encephalopathy and improve cognitive impairment. Highly-active antiretroviral treatment is recommended, preferably including ZDV.

C. Psychostimulants, such as methylphenidate, may improve cognitive performance. The initial dosage is 5 mg orally twice a day.

D. **Olanzapine (Zyprexa)** (2.5 mg bid or 5mg qhs, increasing to 10 to 20 mg qhs if necessary), or risperidone (Risperdal) (starting at 0.5 mg bid, increasing up to 3 mg bid if necessary) may be useful for control of agitation, disinhibition, or psychosis. Neuroleptics can be augmented with lorazepam, 0.5 mg 2 to 3 times daily.

E. **Fluoxetine (Prozac) or Venlafaxine (Effexor XR)**, stimulating antidepressants, are is often effective for apathy accompanying dementia. Methylphenidate (Ritalin), 5 mg twice a day, may also reduce apathy.

III. Depression

A. Major depressive disorder is a common psychiatric diagnosis in HIV-infected patients. Symptoms include depressed mood, changes in sleep and/or appetite and weight, fatigue, loss of interest or pleasure in daily activities, psychomotor slowing or agitation, feelings of worthlessness or guilt, poor concentration, indecisiveness, and recurrent thoughts of death or suicide.

B. Treatment with a selective serotonin reuptake inhibitor (SSRI), such as fluoxetine (Prozac), sertraline (Zoloft), paroxetine (Paxil), or fluvoxamine (Luvox) is recommended. SSRIs are very safe in overdose and lack the anticholinergic and orthostatic side effects of tricyclic antidepressants (TCAs). Initial treatment consists of 10 mg of paroxetine or fluoxetine, or 50 mg sertraline, increasing as necessary to 40 mg paroxetine or fluoxetine or 200 mg sertraline.

C. SSRIs are generally well tolerated, but they may cause nausea, jitteriness, weight loss, insomnia, and sexual dysfunction. These side effects frequently diminish if dosage is reduced or with time.

D. **Bupropion (Wellbutrin)** is a stimulating antidepressant, without the sexual dysfunction of SSRI's, but with a small risk of seizures. The slow release form (Wellbutrin SR) has reduced seizure risk, and is well tolerated. Wellbutrin SR (dose 100 to 200 mg bid) is often used in SSRI nonresponders and in patients who discontinue SSRIs due to sexual dysfunction.

E. **Venlafaxine (Effexor)** has a side effect profile similar to SSRIs, but may be useful in SSRI nonresponders (starting dose 37.5 bid, or 75 mg qd of the slow release form, Effexor XR).

F. **Tricyclic antidepressant agents** are useful for treating peripheral neuropathy pain and depression. They may be effective for those patients who cannot tolerate or who do not respond to SSRIs. TCAs with greater anticholinergic and orthostatic side effects (amitriptyline [Elavil]) should be avoided. A TCA with lower incidence of side effects, such as desipramine (Norpramin) and nortriptyline (Pamelor), is recommended. Side effects of TCAs may include dry mouth, constipation, urinary retention, orthostatic hypotension, increased heart rate, and cognitive impairment. TCAs may cause lethal cardiac effects on overdose.

G. **Nortriptyline (Pamelor)** is mildly sedating; dosage is 50 to 150 mg at bedtime. Desipramine (Norpramin) is somewhat stimulating; its 100- to 300-mg dose may be taken either in the morning or at bedtime.

H. **Insomnia** associated with depression often responds to trazodone (Desyrel, 50 mg every night, increasing if necessary to 150 to 300 mg every night). Side effects of morning grogginess and orthostatic hypotension. In depressed patients with persistent insomnia, trazodone should be used at bedtime in conjunction with a morning dose of fluoxetine, sertraline, or paroxetine.

I. **Apathetic withdrawal** in patients with advanced HIV disease may improve with methylphenidate (Ritalin), 5 mg twice a day. §

References: See page 81.

Wasting

Wasting syndrome is characterized by weight loss of at least 10% for at least 30 days that is not attributable to a concurrent condition other than HIV infection itself. Weight loss has a negative impact on survival and disease progression in AIDS. The prevalence of wasting has declined significantly since the introduction of protease inhibitors.

I. **Clinical evaluation of wasting**
   A. **Body mass index** (BMI; weight in kg divided by height in square meters) is a simple means of comparing a patient's current weight with population norms. Ideal weight for height in adults can be calculated as follows: for men, 106 lbs. for the first 5 feet plus 6 lbs. for each additional inch; for women, 100 lbs. for the first 5 feet plus 5 lbs. for each additional inch.
   B. **Malabsorption** should be excluded as a cause of weight loss because this disorder can occur in the absence of diarrhea. Hypogonadism may be present in men with wasting; therefore, serum testosterone levels should be measured. Free testosterone levels are more accurate than total testosterone levels.
   C. **Dietary assessment** should include a diet history, estimation of current energy intake, and identification of factors that might interfere with food intake. Quantitative estimation of daily intake of energy should be obtained, using techniques such as diet history, 24-hour recall, or prospective food intake diaries.

II. **Treatment of wasting**
   A. **Treatment of underlying disorders,** such as oral or esophageal candidiasis, aphthous ulcers, chronic diarrhea or malabsorption and depression, may result in weight gain.
   B. **Target energy intakes** are 33 to 44 kcal/kg in men and 29 to 44 kcal/kg in women. Protein intake of 1.5 g/kg, a daily multivitamin and a mineral supplement should be recommended.
   C. **Oral nutritional supplementation** can usually increase net daily energy intake. Liquid and solid oral supplements are available.
   D. **Enteral and parenteral feeding.** Repletion or maintenance of weight by enteral or parenteral routes may be considered in individuals who are unable to meet nutritional goals with oral intake.
   E. **Pharmacologic treatments**
      1. **Megestrol acetate (Megace)** is a synthetic progestational agent that may increase food intake and weight; however, weight gain usually consists of fat. Patients treated with 800 mg of megestrol acetate per day for 12 weeks gain an average of 3.5 kg, but gained only 1.1 kg of LBM.
      2. **Dronabinol (Marinol)**
         a. Dronabinol is the synthetic form of tetrahydrocannabinol, the active ingredient in marijuana. Dronabinol consistently improves appetite, but usually provides no weight increase.
         b. This drug is approved for the treatment of HIV-associated anorexia. Side effects include euphoria, dizziness, and thinking abnormalities.
      3. **Recombinant human growth hormone** (rhGH) is effective in producing weight gain and retention of nitrogen and potassium. Side effects included arthralgias, myalgia, puffiness, and diarrhea. It is approved for HIV-associated wasting at a dose of 6 mg/day. Cost

has limited accessibility for many patients.

4. **Anabolic steroids**
   a. **Testosterone replacement** in hypogonadal men increases weight. Testosterone enanthate or cypionate is administered by intramuscular injection (200-400 mg IM 1-2 times per month). Two transdermal preparations are also available.
   b. **Oxandrolone (Oxandrin)** is an oral testosterone derivative that is approved as a treatment for weight loss. A dosage of 5 to 20 mg/day may provide a 0.6 kg weight increase.
   c. **Oxymetholone (Anadrol-50)**, 1 to 2 mg/kg/day, an oral agent, produced a mean weight gain of 5.7 kg and improvements in Karnofsky score in patients with HIV-associated weight loss.
5. **Thalidomide**. In patients with HIV-associated wasting, thalidomide (100 mg four times daily for 12 weeks) produced a median weight gain of 4.05 kg. Patients treated with 100 mg nightly for 8 weeks experienced a 4% increase in weight. Because of teratogenic effects in infants, women of childbearing potential must be advised to use at least two methods of contraception while using thalidomide.

F. **Exercise**. Inactivity is associated with significant loss of muscle mass. Progressive resistance training may increase upper and lower body strength and weight. Combinations of aerobic and resistance training in individuals with HIV infection results in increased fitness level. §

References: See page 81.

HIV Infection in Women

The fastest-growing group becoming infected with HIV is women in their childbearing years, and nearly all children with the infection acquire it perinatally. Women account for 15% of total AIDS cases and for 20% of new cases. AIDS now represents the third most common cause of death in young women overall and the leading cause of death in young African-American women. In over half of HIV-infected women, the infection was acquired through heterosexual contact. Gynecologic complications of HIV infection include a high incidence of abnormal findings on Pap smear, severe pelvic inflammatory disease, breast cancer, and recurrent or persistent vaginal fungal infections.

I. **Cervical disorders**
   A. Human Papilloma Virus and Cervical Neoplasia. Cervical cancer has an increased occurrence and aggressiveness in women with HIV infection. Cervical cancer constitutes an AIDS diagnosis. HPV is an etiologic factor in human and cervical cancer .
   B. Immune suppression increases susceptibility to infection by HPV. HPV prevalence, acquisition, and retention are higher in HIV-positive women. The frequency of abnormal Papanicolaou smear results is increased in HIV-infected women. Squamous intraepithelial lesions have a prevalence of 40% in HIV-positive women.
   C. Because CIN is more frequent and more aggressive in women with severe immunosuppression, a Pap smear should be obtained every 6 months, particularly for women with more advanced immunodeficiency.
   D. Performing a Pap screening every 6 months along with careful vulvar, vaginal, and anal inspection is recommended, especially with more immunosuppressed patients with T cells less than 200 cells/mm^3. Colposcopic evaluation of women should be performed with any atypical squamous cells of unknown significance (ASCUS), atypical glandular cells of unknown significance, low-grade and high-grade SIL on any Pap smear, or any persistent inflammation that is unresolved after treatment for GC, Trichomonas, or Chlamydia.

II. **Vaginal candidiasis**
   A. Vaginal candidiasis, a frequent disorder in women in the general population, may be a source of morbidity for HIV-infected women. Severe vaginal candidiasis is a designated HIV-associated symptomatic disorder.
   B. Vaginal candidiasis may occur in early or late HIV disease, but many women with severe immunosuppression do not have Candida vaginitis.

III. **HIV transmission to the infant**
   A. Zidovudine (Retrovir) administration during pregnancy, labor, delivery, and (administered to the infant) the newborn period reduces the transmission of HIV to 8%, compared with 25% in untreated patients.
   B. **After delivery**, breast-feeding increases risk of transmission of HIV from mothers to infants by about 10% to 19%. Therefore, HIV-infected women are advised against breast-feeding.
   C. **Considerations for antiretroviral therapy in the HIV-infected pregnant woman**
      1. ZDV and 3TC have been evaluated in infected pregnant women, and both appear to be well tolerated and cross the placenta, achieving concentrations in cord blood similar to those observed in maternal blood at delivery. All the nucleosides except ddI pose a potential fetal

   risk and have been classified as pregnancy category C agents; ddI has been classified as category B.

2. ZDV has been shown to reduce the risk of perinatal HIV transmission when administered orally after 14 weeks gestation and continued throughout pregnancy, intravenously administered during the intrapartum period, and to the newborn for the first 6 weeks of life. This chemoprophylactic regimen was shown to reduce the risk of perinatal transmission by 66%. ZDV dosage is 200 mg three times daily or 300 mg twice daily.

3. Monotherapy with ZDV for chemoprophylaxis during pregnancy should be considered for women with CD4$^+$ counts >500/mm^3 and plasma HIV RNA less than 10,000–20,000 RNA copies/mL. For women with more advanced disease and/or higher levels of HIV RNA, a combination antiretroviral regimen that includes ZDV should be given.

4. Monitoring and use of HIV-1 RNA for therapeutic decision-making during pregnancy should be performed as recommended for non-pregnant individuals. Chemoprophylaxis should include intravenous ZDV during delivery and administration of ZDV to the infant for the first six weeks of life. §

References: See page 81.

Opportunistic Infections

Candidiasis

Mucocutaneous candidiasis is the most frequently occurring opportunistic illness in persons with AIDS. Clinical presentations include oropharyngeal candidiasis, esophageal candidiasis, and vulvovaginal candidiasis.

I. **Clinical presentation**
   A. **Oropharyngeal candidiasis** (OPC) causes symptoms of burning pain, altered taste sensation, and difficulty swallowing. Many patients are asymptomatic. Most persons with OPC present with pseudomembranous candidiasis or thrush (white plaques on the buccal mucosa, gums, or tongue) and less commonly with erythematous candidiasis or leukoplakia involving the tongue or angular cheilitis.
   B. **Esophageal candidiasis** is usually accompanied by oropharyngeal candidiasis. Typically, dysphagia and odynophagia are described.
   C. **Vulvovaginal candidiasis** generally presents with itching, watery to cottage cheese-thick discharge, vaginal erythema with adherent white discharge, dyspareunia, external dysuria, erythema, and swelling of labia and vulva with discrete pustulopapular peripheral lesions.

II. **Diagnosis**
   A. The diagnosis of OPC is usually made by its characteristic clinical appearance. The diagnosis of OPC can be confirmed by examining a 10% potassium hydroxide (KOH) slide preparation of a scraping of a lesion. Pseudohyphae and budding yeast are characteristic findings.
   B. A presumptive diagnosis of Cancida esophagitis can be made in a patient with dysphagia and/or odynophagia who has OPC. Upper GI endoscopy can confirm esophageal involvement.
   C. The diagnosis of Candida vaginitis is made by the presence of a characteristic clinical appearance and observation of yeast forms on KOH preparation.

III. **Therapy**
   A. Clotrimazole (Nystatin) is available as an oral spray, solution, and troche. Ketoconazole (Nizoral) is available as a tablet or cream. Oral absorption is enhanced when the gastric pH is less than 4.0. Achlorhydria may interfere with ketoconazole absorption.
   B. Itraconazole (Sporanox), 100 mg qd, is an oral triazole compound, which is available in a suspension, capsule, and parenteral form. Absorption is improved when taken after a full meal.
   C. Fluconazole (Diflucan), 100 mg PO qd, is more completely absorbed than itraconazole or ketoconazole because absorption is not dependent on gastric acidity or food intake.
   D. Esophageal candidiasis requires systemic therapy. Fluconazole (Diflucan), 200 mg PO qd, is more effective than ketoconazole. Itraconazole solution is probably equivalent to fluconazole.
   E. For vulvovaginal candidiasis, topical therapy for 3 days is effective. Agents include clotrimazole (Gyne-Lotrimin) and Miconazole (Monistat 3) cream. A one-time dose of 150 mg of fluconazole is highly effective.

IV. **Refractory candidiasis**
   A. Persons with OPC that is unresponsive to clotrimazole, ketoconazole, or itraconazole tablets will usually respond to fluconazole. Persons with

OPC unresponsive to fluconazole (200 mg daily given for 2 weeks) may respond to higher doses of fluconazole. For fluconazole-refractory OPC, amphotericin B oral suspension (100 mg po qid) or itraconazole (100 mg qd) may be effective.

B. Treatment duration is 7 to 14 days for OPC or vaginal disease and up to 21 days for esophageal disease. §

References: See page 81.

Pneumocystis Carinii Pneumonia

PCP is the most common life-threatening opportunistic infection occurring in patients with HIV disease. In the era of PCP prophylaxis and highly-active antiretroviral therapy, the incidence of PCP is decreasing. The incidence of PCP has declined steadily from 50% in 1987 to 25% currently.

I. **Risk factors for Pneumocystis carinii pneumonia**
   A. Patients with CD4 counts of 200 cells/μL or less are 4.9 times more likely to develop PCP compared with patients with CD4 counts of more than 200 cells/μL.
   B. Candidates for PCP prophylaxis include: patients with a prior history of PCP, patients with a CD4 cell count of less than 200 cells/μL, and HIV-infected patients with thrush or persistent fevers.

II. **Clinical presentation**
   A. PCP usually presents with fever, dry cough, and shortness of breath or dyspnea on exertion with a gradual onset over several weeks. Physical findings are often minimal; however, tachypnea may be pronounced, and patients may be so dyspneic that they are unable to speak without stopping to rest. Circumoral, acral, and mucous membrane cyanosis may be evident.
   B. **Laboratory findings**
      1. **Complete blood counts and sedimentation rates** show no characteristic pattern in patients with PCP. Serum chemistries are not particularly helpful; however, the serum LDH concentration is frequently increased.
      2. **Arterial blood gas** measurements generally show increases in P(A-a)O$_2$, although PaO$_2$ values vary widely depending on disease severity. Up to 25% of patients may have a PaO2 of 80 mm Hg or above while breathing room air.
      3. **Pulmonary function tests**. Patients with PCP usually have a decrease in diffusing capacity for carbon monoxide (DLCO).
   C. **Radiographic presentation**
      1. PCP in AIDS patients usually causes a diffuse interstitial infiltrate. High resolution computerized tomography (HRCT) may be helpful for those patients who have normal chest radiographic findings.
      2. Pneumatoceles (cavities, cysts, blebs, or bullae) and spontaneous pneumothoraces in patients with PCP are common.

III. **Laboratory diagnosis**
   A. **Sputum induction.** The least invasive means of establishing a specific diagnosis is the examination of sputum induced by inhalation of a 3 to 5% saline mist. The sensitivity of induced sputum examination for PCP is 74 to 77% and the negative predictive value is 58 to 64%. If the sputum tests negative, an invasive diagnostic procedure is required to confirm the diagnosis of PCP.
   B. **Transbronchial biopsy and bronchoalveolar lavage.** The sensitivity of transbronchial biopsy for PCP is 98%. The sensitivity of bronchoalveolar is 90%.
   C. **Open lung biopsy** should be reserved for patients with progressive pulmonary disease in whom the less invasive procedures are nondiagnostic.

IV. Diagnostic algorithm

A. If the chest radiograph of a symptomatic patient appears normal, a DLCO should be performed. Patients with significant symptoms, a normal-appearing chest radiograph, and a normal DLCO should undergo high-resolution CT. Patients with abnormal findings at any of these steps should proceed to sputum induction or bronchoscopy. Sputum specimens collected by induction that reveal P. carinii should also be stained for acid-fast organisms and fungi, and the specimen should be cultured for mycobacteria and fungi.

B. Patients whose sputum examinations do not show P. carinii or another pathogen should undergo bronchoscopy.

C. Lavage fluid is stained for P. carinii, acid-fast organisms, and fungi. Also, lavage fluid is cultured for mycobacteria and fungi and inoculated onto cell culture for viral isolation. Touch imprints are made from tissue specimens and stained for P. carinii. Tissue is cultured for mycobacteria and fungi, and stained for P. carinii, acid-fast organisms, and fungi. If all procedures are nondiagnostic and the lung disease is progressive, clinicians open lung biopsy may be considered.

V. Therapy and prophylaxis

A. Trimethoprim-sulfamethoxazole (Bactrim, Septra) is the recommended initial therapy for PCP. Dosage is 15 mg/kg/day of TMP and 75 mg/kg/day of SMX divided every 8 hours for 14 to 21 days. Adverse effects include rash (33%), elevation of liver enzymes (44%), nausea and vomiting (50%), anemia (40%), creatinine elevation (33%), and hyponatremia (94%). The most common adverse reactions that necessitated a change in therapy were neutropenia (15%) and severe rash (15%).

B. Pentamidine is an alternative in patients who have adverse reactions or fail to respond to TMP-SMX. The dosage is 3 mg/kg/day for 14 to 21 days. Adverse effects include anemia (33%), creatinine elevation (60%), LFT elevation (63%), and hyponatremia (56%). The most common adverse effect requiring a change in therapy is neutropenia (32%). Pancreatitis, hypoglycemia, and hyperglycemia are common side effects of pentamidine. Hypoglycemia or hyperglycemia occurs in 57% of all patients.

C. Corticosteroids. Adjunctive corticosteroid treatment is beneficial with anti-PCP therapy in patients with a partial pressure of oxygen (PaO_2) less than 70 mm Hg, $(A-a)DO_2$ greater than 35 mm Hg, or oxygen saturation less than 90% on room air. Contraindications include suspected tuberculosis or disseminated fungal infection. Treatment with prednisone (40 mg twice daily for 5 days, then 40 mg daily for 5 days, and then 20 mg daily until day 21 of therapy) should begin at the same time as anti-PCP therapy.

VI. Prophylaxis

A. PCP is the most common life-threatening opportunistic infection in HIV-infected patients. HIV-infected patients who have CD4 counts less than 200 cells per microliter or who have survived an episode of PCP should receive prophylaxis against PCP.

B. Trimethoprim-sulfamethoxazole (once daily to thrice weekly) is the preferred regimen for PCP prophylaxis because of efficacy and simultaneous efficacy in prophylaxis against toxoplasmosis.

C. Dapsone (100 mg daily or twice weekly) is a prophylactic regimen for patients who can not tolerate TMP-SMX. Adverse reactions included anemia, LDH elevation, methemoglobinemia, nausea, and skin rash. §

References: See page 81.

Bacterial Infections Associated with HIV Disease

Bacterial infections are a common cause of death in HIV-infected patients. HIV-infected patients may not present with an acute onset of symptoms, fever, or elevated white blood cell count, which are characteristic of bacterial infections in the normal host.

I. **Haemophilus influenzae**
    A. Haemophilus influenzae is one of the most common bacterial infections occurring in persons infected with HIV. HIV infection increases the risk of acquiring H. influenzae infection.
    B. Pneumonia, sepsis, and, less often, meningitis are the clinical syndromes most frequently seen. Fever and productive cough suggest pneumonia. Meningitis usually presents with meningismus and fever.
    C. Most patients have an elevated white blood cell count, with a left shift in 65%. Cultures of blood, CSF, or joint fluid confirm the diagnosis. A positive sputum culture alone should be interpreted with caution as H. influenzae can colonize the pharynx. Positive blood cultures are found in 20% of adults with H. influenzae pneumonia. Chest radiographs most commonly reveal unilateral or bilateral infiltrates.
    D. **Treatment**. A third generation cephalosporin, trimethoprim-sulfamethoxazole, or a second generation cephalosporin are recommended until identification and sensitivities of the organism have been determined. Because chest radiographs can mimic PCP pneumonia, empiric treatment for bacterial pneumonia and PCP should be initiated until a definitive diagnosis is made.

II. **Pseudomonas aeruginosa**
    A. P. aeruginosa is an important opportunistic pathogens in the HIV-infected host. Risk factors include recent hospitalization; catheters; neutropenia; cytomegalovirus infection; prior PCP; aerosolized pentamidine; recent antimicrobial, antiviral or immunosuppressive therapy; and steroids.
    B. Manifestations include pneumonia, sepsis, catheter-associated bacteremia, urinary tract infection, meningitis, malignant otitis externa, endocarditis, corneal and conjunctival ulcers, sinusitis, osteomyelitis, septic arthritis, and soft tissue infections. The majority of HIV-infected persons with P. aeruginosa infections have low CD4 counts (<100) and a previous or concomitant AIDS-defining illness. Pneumonia and bacteremia are the most common syndromes in HIV-infected persons. Fever and productive cough are typically present.
    C. **Diagnosis**. Bacteremia is seen in 25 to 56% of cases of pneumonia. Sputum cultures are positive in 54 to 100% of cases of pneumonia. Chest radiographs usually reveal focal infiltrates; cavities may be seen in 69%.
    D. **Combination therapy** with an antipseudomonal beta lactam plus an aminoglycoside is recommended.

III. **Rhodococcus equi**
    A. **Epidemiology.** Rhodococcus equi is a gram-positive aerobic pleomorphic coccobacillus. In AIDS patients with R. equi infection, the average CD4 count is 50 cells/μL.

B. Pneumonia is the most common manifestation of R. equi infection, manifesting as fever, cough, pleuritic chest pain, and dyspnea; hemoptysis and weight loss may also occur. Subcutaneous, renal, pelvic, brain abscesses, osteomyelitis, mycetoma, and post-traumatic endophthalmitis may also occur.

C. A history of exposure to farm animals or manure may or may not be present. Chest radiographs may reveal consolidation (without lobar predilection), cavities (in 75%), mass lesions, or pleural effusions (18-35%). Sputum and blood cultures will be positive for R. equi in 50%. Bronchoscopy or biopsy may be necessary when all cultures are sterile. Acid-fast smears are variably positive and may be misinterpreted as tuberculosis or other mycobacteria.

D. Treatment and Outcome

    1. Vancomycin plus imipenem has been effective. Antimicrobial susceptibility testing must guide the choice of antibiotics. At least two antibiotics to which R. equi is sensitive should be used.

    2. Initial therapy should be given for at least 2 months, preferably with intravenous antibiotics. Maintenance therapy should be given for life with two antibiotics to which the organism is known to be susceptible.

IV. Salmonellae

A. Salmonellae can cause gastroenteritis, enteric fever, and focal infections. Poultry, eggs and unpasteurized milk are the largest sources of human infection. Person-to-person transmission can also occur via the fecal-oral route.

B. Salmonella infections in AIDS patients usually manifest as severe gastroenteritis, bacteremia, or extraintestinal focal infection. Patients present with diarrhea, fever, and bacteremia. Salmonella may be isolated in blood and/or stool cultures.

C. Treatment. Ceftriaxone (Rocephin), 1 to 2 g IV q 24 hours, and ciprofloxacin (Cipro), 750 mg PO bid, have been shown to be effective.

§

References: See page 81.

Toxoplasmosis

Toxoplasma gondii, an obligate intracellular protozoan, is a major cause of morbidity and mortality among patients with advanced HIV disease. The cat is a major vector in transmission. Excretion of oocysts occurs in 1% of cats, although cockroaches and flies can also transmit the infection. Transmission to humans usually occurs by the oral route (eating poorly cooked meat or contaminated food). T. gondii can cause acute, latent, and reactivated disease.

I. **Epidemiology**. Ten to 50% of adults in the United States are Toxoplasma gondii seropositive. HIV-infected persons have a high incidence of reactivation disease. Thirty to 40% of AIDS patients who are seropositive for Toxoplasma develop active toxoplasmosis as a result of reactivation of their latent infection.

II. **Clinical presentation**
   A. Headache, usually dull and constant, occurs in about 50% of patients presenting with Toxoplasma encephalitis (TE).
   B. Fever occurs in 40 to 50% of cases of TE, and confusion and lethargy are common. Frank meningismus occurs in 5% of patients, and 15 to 30% present with seizures. Seizures in an HIV-infected patient are usually caused by toxoplasmosis. At the time of physical examination, up to 75% of patients are found to have focal neurologic deficits.
   C. **CNS toxoplasmosis** of causes about 50 to 70% of focal CNS deficits in patients with advanced HIV disease; the remainder are caused by primary CNS lymphoma (20 to 30%) and progressive multifocal leukoencephalopathy (PML) (10 to 20%).

III. **Diagnostic evaluation**
   A. **Head CT scan** in patients with CNS toxoplasmosis reveals enhancing lesions, usually in the form of ring enhancement, in 80 to 90% of patients. About 60 to 70% of patients have multiple lesions by CT or MRI. Lesions are most common in the frontal lobes, basal ganglia, and parietal lobes, and generally in cerebral white matter or subcortical gray matter.
   B. **MRI** is more sensitive than CT in detecting intracranial pathology. MRI should be the initial neuroimaging procedure for HIV-infected patients with neurologic symptoms. Neither CT nor MRI is definitive for securing the diagnosis of TE because CNS lymphoma and other infectious processes can have a similar radiologic appearance.
   C. **Lumbar puncture** excludes other opportunistic infections as the cause of neurologic signs and symptoms, such as meningitides caused by Cryptococcus or M. tuberculosis. If focal neurologic deficits or clinical evidence of increased intracranial pressure are present, a CT or MRI should be completed before lumbar puncture.
   D. **Cerebrospinal fluid** (CSF) analysis in patients with toxoplasmic encephalitis usually reveals a normal glucose level. Protein levels are slightly elevated in half of patients. A mild mononuclear pleocytosis is present in 15 to 50%.
   E. **Serologic Diagnosis**
      1. AIDS-associated TE is most often due to reactivation of latent toxoplasmosis. Serum IgG titers are positive in 80 to 90% of patients.
      2. IgG titer should be measured for all HIV-infected patients early in their disease because a positive serologic finding, regardless of titer, indicates that the patient is at risk for reactivation of latent

toxoplasmosis. Up to 40% of HIV-positive patients with positive IgG anti-Toxoplasma antibodies develop active CNS toxoplasmosis within 2 years after the onset of AIDS.

3. In patients who have signs and symptoms suggestive of reactivated toxoplasmosis, toxoplasmosis titer should be determined if the patient has never had a titer measured in the past, because a negative IgG titer is uncommon in a patient with reactivated toxoplasmosis.

IV. Treatment of toxoplasmosis

A. Acute treatment

1. HIV-infected patients with TE should be treated for 8 weeks or until all CT evidence of toxoplasmosis has resolved. A follow-up imaging study should be completed after 2 weeks of treatment.

2. **Sulfadiazine and pyrimethamine combination regimen**

   a. **Sulfadiazine**

      (1) The initial dose of sulfadiazine is 1.0 to 1.5 g orally every 6 hours. Side effects include neutropenia, nausea, vomiting, diarrhea, rash, fever, interstitial nephritis, crystalluria, and nephrolithiasis.

      (2) Patients should drink 2 to 3 liters of fluid per day because dehydration increases the risk of crystallization of sulfadiazine in the urinary collecting system.

   b. **Pyrimethamine.** The initial dose of pyrimethamine is a 200 mg PO followed by 50 to 100 mg PO per day. Side effects include pancytopenia, headache, and gastrointestinal upset. To decrease the incidence of pancytopenia, 10 mg of folinic acid is administered orally with each dose of pyrimethamine.

B. Maintenance therapy for chronic suppression of toxoplasmosis

1. HIV-infected patients with TE require suppressive anti-Toxoplasma therapy for life. The first choice for maintenance therapy is sulfadiazine (2 to 4 g/day in four divided doses) along with pyrimethamine (25 to 50 mg/day) and folinic acid (10 mg/day).

C. Prevention of toxoplasmosis in HIV-infected persons

1. **Prevention of seroconversion.** HIV-infected persons with a cat who are seronegative for Toxoplasma should change their cat litter boxes daily so that oocysts are discarded before they mature; they should cook meats thoroughly (reaching internal temperatures of 66°C for at least 10 minutes); and wash their hands after contact with soil.

2. **Prevention of reactivation disease in seropositives.** Chemoprophylaxis is recommended for all HIV-infected persons who are seropositive for Toxoplasma and who have CD4 counts below 100 cells/μL. Oral sulfamethoxazole-trimethoprim is the preferred regimen (one double-strength tablet daily to one double-strength tablet twice weekly). Oral dapsone (100 mg twice weekly) and pyrimethamine (25 mg twice weekly) is a second-line alternative. §

References: See page 81.

Mycobacterium Tuberculosis Infection

Tuberculosis (TB) is a frequent and treatable cause of morbidity and mortality in HIV-infected patients. Most cases are caused by reactivation of dormant TB infection secondary to decreased cell-mediated immunity. *M. tuberculosis* is transmitted by respiratory droplets spread by by coughing, sneezing, or talking. The infectious droplets may remain airborne for up to 48 hours.

I. Clinical presentation
    A. **In patients with earlier stages of HIV disease** (CD4 cell counts of 300 cells/mm^3 or above), the presentation tends to be like that in persons without immunodeficiency. A productive cough of several weeks duration, hemoptysis, fever, and weight loss are common. Chest x-ray reveals focal infiltrates and cavities involving the upper lobes.
    B. **In patients with more pronounced immunodeficiency** (CD4 counts of less than 200 cells/mm^3) the features of TB tend to be atypical, with greater frequency of extrapulmonary involvement and diffuse pulmonary disease without cavitation.
    C. **Patients with advanced HIV disease** more often have miliary TB and involvement of the lymphatic system, central nervous system (parenchymal and meningeal), soft tissue, bone marrow, liver, and other viscera. Fever is common, but cough may not be present. There may be a prior history of TB. Chest x-ray may demonstrate involvement of any lobe of the lungs, and the clinical presentation may be indistinguishable from a community-acquired pneumonia. Cervical, hilar, paratracheal, or mediastinal adenopathy are highly suggestive of TB.

II. Diagnosis
    A. **Tuberculin skin testing** is positive in only 30 to 50% of HIV-infected patients with tuberculosis react to the. Chest radiographs may not show classic upper-lobe infiltrates. Diffuse, interstitial, or lower-lobe infiltrates, often with prominent hilar and paratracheal enlargement, are common findings.
    B. **Sputum acid-fast bacilli (AFB) smears** are positive in half of patients. Ninety percent of cases of pulmonary tuberculosis will be identified by examination of three expectorated or induced sputum specimens obtained on separate days for smear and culture for AFB. Because failure to identify AFB on smear may occur, diagnosis may require repeated culture of specimens from bone marrow, lymph nodes, brain tissue, cerebrospinal fluid, urine, stool, or blood.
    C. If TB is strongly suspected, empiric therapy should be initiated while awaiting culture results. Because the sensitivity of culture is 90%, negative cultures do not guarantee the absence of TB.
    D. **Rapid detection methods**, the Amplicor PCR and Amplified Mycobacterium Tuberculosis Direct Test ([AMTD], Gen-Probe), can be used in identification of *M. tuberculosis* in smear-positive sputum specimens. These methods are more sensitive than acid-fast staining, but are slightly less sensitive than culture, which remains the gold standard. Rapid tests should not be used to confirm or exclude the diagnosis of TB except in cases in which smears reveal acid-fast bacteria.
    E. Diagnosis or treatment of TB can be accomplished in the outpatient setting. Once a diagnosis of TB is made or appears likely, contact investigation should be initiated (for confirmed cases) and exposure of

additional persons should be prevented.

III. Treatment

A. Patients with HIV disease who have positive findings on AFB smears of sputum or biopsy specimens, or whose cultures yield an acid-fast organism, should be treated for *M. tuberculosis* pending final culture results. If sputum smears do not reveal AFB, but active TB is suspected in an HIV-infected patient, empiric therapy should be initiated pending culture results. In some cases, *Mycobacterium avium* complex (MAC) infection will be the final diagnosis.

Antituberculous Agents, Ranked in Order of Preference, Usual Daily Dose, and Principle Toxicities

Drug	Daily Dose	Principal Route	Toxicities
First line drugs			
Isoniazid	300 mg	po or im	Hepatitis, neuritis
Rifampin	600 mg	po or iv	Hepatitis, drug interactions
Ethambutol	1 5 - 2 5 mg/kg	po	Optic neuritis (at higher doses)
Pyrazinamide	25 mg/kg	po	Hyperuricemia, hepatitis
Second line drugs			
Streptomycin	15 mg/kg	im	Ototoxicity and vestibulotoxicity with renal insufficiency
Ofloxacin	400 mg bid	po	Gastrointestinal
Ciprofloxacin	750 mg bid	po	Gastrointestinal
Amikacin	15 mg/kg	im	Same as streptomycin
Capreomycin	15 mg/kg	im	Same as streptomycin
Kanamycin	15 mg/kg	im	Same as streptomycin, but more toxic
Ethionamide	0.5 - 1.0 g	po	Gastrointestinal, hepatitis
Cycloserine	0.5 - 1.0 g	po	Neuropsychiatric
Clofazimine	2 0 0 - 3 0 0 mg	po	Dark skin
Rifabutin	300 mg	po	Drug interactions, uveitis, rash
Para-aminosalicylic acid (PAS)	8-12 g	po	Gastrointestinal, rash

B. The recommended initial treatment regimen for patients with HIV infection and TB consists of 2 months of daily isoniazid (INH), rifampin, pyrazinamide, and ethambutol, followed by 4 to 7 months of daily or

twice-weekly INH and rifampin.
- C. **Interactions between rifamycins and Protease Inhibitors.**
    1. Rifamycins (rifampin) are inducers of cytochrome P450 enzymes. Because protease inhibitors are metabolized by this enzyme system, the concentration of protease inhibitor is likely to be subtherapeutic with concomitant administration of a rifamycin. Ritonavir and indinavir also inhibit cytochrome P450 enzymes and decrease metabolism of the rifamycins, which may accumulate to toxic levels.
    2. The antiretroviral regimen should include indinavir (800 mg every 8 hours) as the protease inhibitor, and rifabutin (Mycobutin) (150 mg per day) should be substituted for rifampin in a 9-month treatment regimen.

IV. Monitoring therapy

- A. Response of pulmonary TB to therapy is monitored by following sputum smear and culture results monthly until they become negative. Sputum smears typically become negative after the first month. Cultures should be negative after 2 to 3 months. Positive cultures persisting beyond the third month suggest the possibility of noncompliance with medications, drug resistance, or both. Sputum should also be cultured at 3, 6, and 12 months after therapy is completed to monitor for relapse.
- B. **Criteria for discontinuing isolation**. Once effective chemotherapy has been administered for at least 2 weeks, patients can resume work and social contacts provided that three sputum smears are negative for AFB.

V. Screening and prevention

- A. **Tuberculin skin testing.** All HIV-infected persons should be screened for TB by tuberculin skin testing. When a reaction is ≥ 5 mm in a person who does not have active TB, prophylaxis should be initiated with INH (300 mg per day for 12 months).
- B. **Treatment of contacts**
    1. Patients with HIV disease and TB who have positive findings in sputum or bronchoscopy specimens are infectious and their contacts should be screened for TB and given prophylaxis when indicated. HIV-positive contacts to individuals with active TB should receive INH, even if the contact's PPD skin response is less than 5 mm because the contact may be anergic. Active TB should be excluded before initiating prophylaxis.
    2. HIV-positive contacts to patients with multi-drug resistant TB should receive prophylaxis with two drugs to which the organism from the index patient is susceptible. A 12-month regimen of pyrazinamide 25 mg/kg plus ofloxacin 600 mg once daily is usually effective. §

References: See page 81.

Cytomegalovirus Retinitis

Cytomegalovirus (CMV) is a common opportunistic pathogen in individuals infected with HIV, causing retinitis, colitis, and encephalitis. Cytomegalovirus disease occurs in 20-40% of patients with AIDS. HIV-infected persons with CD4$^+$ cell counts below 50/μL are at highest risk for CMV disease. Retinitis usually begins unilaterally, but, untreated, progression to bilateral involvement is common.

I. **Clinical evaluation**
   A. Retinitis is the most common manifestation of CMV infection, accounting for 75% to 85% of CMV disease. Typically, the disease appears as a yellow to white area of retinal necrosis and edema, which follows a vascular distribution and is sometimes hemorrhagic. An ophthalmologist can establish the diagnosis with a dilated retinal examination.
   B. Symptoms of CMV retinitis may include light flashes, floaters, loss of central or peripheral visual field, and blurred or distorted vision. Asymptomatic retinitis can be detected by ophthalmologic screening of HIV-infected persons at high risk.
   C. Patients with CD4$^+$ cell counts below 50/μL should receive ophthalmologic screening every 3 to 6 months. Patients with extraocular CMV disease should also be examined regularly.

II. **Treatment of cytomegalovirus retinitis**
   A. **Ganciclovir**
      1. Ganciclovir is a nucleoside analogue. Intravenous and oral ganciclovir are available for clinical use. It is administered by intravenous infusion over 1 hour in a dosage of 5 mg/kg two times daily during initial induction (14-21 days). Maintenance therapy consists of 5 mg/kg once daily. The dosage must be reduced with impaired renal function.
      2. Initial response in retinitis occurs in 75% of patients. Maintenance therapy should be continued for life. Even with continued maintenance therapy, progression of CMV retinitis eventually occurs. Maintenance intravenous ganciclovir is given in a dose of 5-6 mg/kg, 5-7 days per week.
      3. Oral treatment (4.5 and 6.0 grams/day) is inferior to intravenous treatment.
      4. **Intravitreal treatment.** Intravitreal delivery is effective and safe, although it does not treat systemic CMV disease that is frequently present in patients with retinitis. Sustained intravitreal release by a surgically implantable device must be accompanied by systemic therapy (eg, oral drug) to prevent contralateral eye and extraocular disease.
      5. **Clinical use of ganciclovir.** Intravenous ganciclovir is recommended for the initial treatment of acute CMV infection. Oral ganciclovir may be considered for maintenance therapy (not induction) in patients who do not have immediate sight-threatening disease (ie, retinitis near the macula or the optic nerve) because it is not as effective as intravenous therapy.
      6. **Resistance.** After 3 months of ganciclovir therapy, 10% of AIDS patients develop resistant CMV. These strains remain sensitive to foscarnet, which may be used as alternate therapy.
      7. **Ganciclovir toxicity** frequently limits therapy with ganciclovir.

Sixteen percent of patients receiving ganciclovir develop neutrophil counts of less than 500/μL. The dosage should be reduced when absolute neutrophil counts fall below 750-1000 μL or discontinued when severe leukopenia occurs (absolute neutrophil counts less than 500/μL). Cytokines such as granulocyte colony-stimulating factor (G-CSF) are effective in reversing ganciclovir-induced neutropenia. Thrombocytopenia occurs in 9%.

B. Foscarnet

1. Foscarnet is a pyrophosphate that inhibits herpes DNA polymerase. Induction therapy is 60 mg/kg administered intravenously every 8 hours. Maintenance dosage is 120 mg/kg.

2. **Adverse effects** include renal impairment, anemia, hypocalcemia, hypomagnesemia, and hypophosphatemia. Daily infusion of a 1 liter saline reduces nephrotoxicity.

C. Combination therapy with ganciclovir and foscarnet is effective for relapsing retinitis in patients initially treated with either ganciclovir or foscarnet. When ganciclovir, 5 mg/kg/day was used together with foscarnet 90 mg/kg/day, the combination therapy controlled CMV retinitis more effectively than ganciclovir or foscarnet alone.

D. Cidofovir

1. Cidofovir is a nucleotide analog, which is active against the majority of ganciclovir-resistant CMV strains. The drug has an extremely long half-life, permitting intravenous administration every 2 weeks during maintenance treatment. Induction therapy consists of 5 mg/kg IV weekly for 2 weeks. Maintenance therapy is 5 mg/kg IV every 2 weeks.

2. Cidofovir is nephrotoxic, but this can be diminished by prehydration and probenecid (2 g PO 3 hours prior to cidofovir, 1 g PO 2 hours after, and 1 g PO 8 hours after). Renal function and toxicity must be monitored carefully, and proteinuria or a rising creatinine are reasons for dosage reduction, interruption, or discontinuation. §

References: See page 81.

Aspergillosis

In AIDS patients, aspergillosis most commonly affects the lungs, causing a thick-walled cavitary disease of the upper lobes, diffuse unilateral of bilateral infiltrates, ulcerative tracheobronchial disease, or obstructive bronchitis. The brain is the second most commonly involved organ. Aspergillus species are ubiquitous throughout the world, growing in decaying vegetation and soil.

I. **Clinical presentation**
   A. Aspergillus infections are relatively uncommon in patients with advanced HIV disease (4%). Most Aspergillus infections occur in patients with coexisting opportunistic infections, neutroperia, or other risk factors.
   B. **Pulmonary involvement** is the most common site of invasive aspergillosis, manifesting as fever, dyspnea, cough, chest pain, and hemoptysis. In one third of patients, chest radiographic findings include thick-walled cavities, most commonly in the upper lobes. Unilateral or bilateral diffuse or nodular infiltrates are visualized in 20% of patients.
   C. **Extrapulmonary involvement** most commonly involves the central nervous system (CNS), causing abscesses and hemorrhagic or mycotic aneurysms. CNS involvement manifests with focal neurologic deficits and other signs attributed to an intracranial mass lesion.

II. **Evaluation**
   A. Sputum, blood, bone marrow, organ tissue may be examined by microscopy and cultured for fungi.
   B. Only 10 to 30% of patients with invasive pulmonary aspergillosis have positive findings on sputum culture. Cultures of bronchoalveolar lavage fluid are positive in most patients with invasive pulmonary aspergillosis. The fungus is rarely cultured from blood, cerebrospinal fluid, bone marrow, or other organs.

III. **Treatment**
   A. **Amphotericin B,** 1.0 mg/kg/day, is the treatment of choice. Amphotericin B in combination with flucytosine has been used.
   B. **Itraconazole (Sporanox),** 300 mg twice daily for 3 days and then 200 mg twice daily for 12 weeks, has activity against Aspergillus; it is active after oral administration and has less adverse effects than amphotericin B. §

References: See page 81.

Cryptococcosis

Cryptococcosis is the most common cause of life-threatening meningitis in AIDS. Approximately 5-8% of patients with AIDS develop cryptococcal infection. Meningoencephalitis is the most frequent manifestation of cryptococcosis in HIV-infected individuals. Cryptococcal pneumonia is the most frequent fungal pneumonia encountered in persons with AIDS, except in areas hyperendemic for either histoplasmosis or coccidioidomycosis. The organism is ubiquitous in the environment, and transmission occurs via the respiratory route.

I. **Clinical presentation**
   - A. **Pulmonary cryptococcosis**. Patients may present with cough, fever, malaise, shortness of breath, and pleuritic pain. Physical examination may reveal lymphadenopathy, tachypnea, and/or crackles. Chest radiographs reveal focal or diffuse infiltrates. Less common chest radiograph findings include solitary subpleural nodules, mass-like infiltrates with consolidation, hilar and mediastinal adenopathy, and pleural effusions.
   - B. **Central nervous system (CNS) cryptococcal invasion**
     1. The CNS is the most common site of disseminated cryptococcal infection. CNS invasion may be secondary to hematogenous infection or may represent reactivation disease. Infection typically presents as headache, fever, and altered mental status. Cranial nerve palsies and papilledema are the most common ocular manifestations. Complications of CNS infection include hydrocephalus, motor or sensory deficits, cerebellar dysfunction, seizures, and dementia.
     2. Opening pressure is greater than 200 mm H_2O in 70% of patients. Computed tomography (CT) or magnetic resonance imaging (MRI) scans may reveal intracerebral granulomata referred to as cryptococcomas.
     3. Abnormal cerebrospinal fluid (CSF) findings, such as a pleocytosis, low glucose concentrations, and high protein concentrations, are seen in 40%. A minimal inflammatory CSF response, characterized by <10 lymphocytes/mm^3, is seen in 55%. Cryptococcal meningitis may present with normal CSF findings in 26%.

II. **Laboratory evaluation**
   - A. **India ink stain** of CSF is positive in over 80% of patients with AIDS. Encapsulated yeasts seen on Alcian blue or mucicarmine or Gomori methenamine silver are diagnostic of cryptococcus.
   - B. **Cryptococcal Antigen**
     1. Cryptococcal antigen in the serum is indicative of systemic disease. Cryptococcal antigen has greater than 95% sensitivity and specificity in the diagnosis of true invasive cryptococcal infection. Serum cryptococcal antigens are 99% positive in cryptococcal meningitis. A negative serum cryptococcal antigen result suggests that the patient is unlikely to have CNS disease.
     2. With management of cryptococcal meningitis, CSF cryptococcal antigen titers should decrease after 2 or more weeks of therapy.

III. **Treatment**
   - A. **Acute infection**
     1. Patients with cryptococcal meningitis should be treated with amphotericin B, 0.7 mg/kg/day, with or without flucytosine, 100 mg/kg/day, followed by 8 weeks of either fluconazole (Diflucan), 400

mg/day, or itraconazole (Sporanox), 400 mg/day.

2. Aggressive management of acute cerebral edema/intracranial pressure is essential. Intracranial pressure should be measured at the time of initial lumbar puncture and again if any clinical deterioration is noted. Daily lumbar punctures, removing approximately 30 ml until the pressure remains decreased, lumbar drains, or ventriculoperitoneal shunts should be considered.

3. **Maintenance therapy.** Patients with AIDS must continue chronic suppressive therapy with fluconazole (200 mg qd) for life. Repeat lumbar punctures should be performed after completion of therapy and at anytime there is clinical evidence to suggest relapse. §

References: See page 81.

Histoplasmosis

Histoplasma capsulatum is endemic to the Mississippi and Ohio River Valleys, the Caribbean, and Central and South America. Both reactivation of previously acquired infections and newly acquired infections can lead to disseminated disease in AIDS patients. In endemic areas, disseminated histoplasmosis is a frequent complication of AIDS.

I. **Clinical presentation**
   A. **Acute Histoplasmosis**. In 40% of patients, the primary infection produces a flu-like illness with fever (95%), anorexia (85%), nonproductive cough (75%), and chest pain (75%). Physical examination usually reveals pulmonary crackles and adenopathy. Scattered infiltrates and hilar adenopathy occur in up to 25% of patients.
   B. **Disseminated Histoplasmosis.** The initial pulmonary infection infrequently progresses to disseminated disease, manifesting as high fever, weight loss, respiratory complaints, hepatomegaly, splenomegaly, lymphadenopathy, pancytopenia, and sepsis with hypotension.
   C. **Chest radiographic findings** of disseminated histoplasmosis include diffuse nodular infiltrates or linear/irregular opacities.

II. **Diagnosis**
   A. In patients with advanced HIV disease and a history of exposure to the fungus in endemic areas, histoplasmosis may cause sepsis, respiratory disease, CNS processes, hepatomegaly and splenomegaly, chronic nonspecific febrile illness, pancytopenia, and chronic wasting syndrome.
   B. Culture of bone marrow biopsy or aspirate specimens, peripheral blood smear (including buffy coat), lymph node biopsy specimens, bronchoalveolar lavage fluid sample, transbronchial biopsy material, and biopsy samples of cutaneous lesions are usually diagnostic. Blood and urine should be cultured for fungi.
   C. Serologic tests that detect antibodies against histoplasma antigens are not reliable for definitive diagnosis because they lack sensitivity and specificity; however, a fourfold rise in titer is significant.
   D. Skin testing with histoplasmin has no role in the diagnosis of histoplasmosis. More than 50% of the population residing in an endemic area may have positive skin tests. The skin test is negative in 50% of patients with disseminated histoplasmosis.

III. **Treatment**
   A. **Initial therapy**
      1. Amphotericin B is the treatment of choice for HIV-infected patients with moderate to severe disseminated disease or who have either endocarditis or CNS involvement. The initial dose is 1 mg/kg/day to a cumulative dose of 15 to 30 mg/kg. Liposomal amphotericin B may be useful for patients at increased risk for amphotericin B nephrotoxicity.
      2. Itraconazole (Sporanox) is an alternative to amphotericin B for the treatment of mild disseminated histoplasmosis in AIDS patients; 300 mg twice daily for 3 days and then 200 mg twice daily for 12 weeks.
   B. **Maintenance Therapy**. Lifelong suppressive therapy is recommended because of relapse rates of 50 to 90%. Itraconazole is the preferred oral drug for chronic suppressive therapy for histoplasmosis; 200-400 mg qd. Fluconazole is less effective than itraconazole. In patients who cannot

tolerate itraconazole, fluconazole (200-400 mg per day orally) is a reasonable alternative.

References: See page 81.

Coccidioidomycosis

Coccidioidomycosis is a fungal infection endemic to the southwestern United States, Mexico, and Central and South America. Acute infection presents as a flu-like syndrome, a severe pneumonia, or rarely, disseminated disease and death. The acute disease typically resolves spontaneously, but in some patients, it progresses to chronic localized disease of the lungs or other organs such as bone, skin, and meninges. Infection with C. immitis can disseminate in patients with HIV infection. Patients with AIDS most commonly develop diffuse reticulonodular pulmonary disease.

I. **Clinical presentation**
   A. **Acute pulmonary infection**. Only about 40% of patients acutely infected with C. immitis experience a flu-like syndrome with chest pain and cough. Chest radiographs may show single or multiple nodules, thin-walled cavities, hilar or mediastinal lymphadenopathy, or pneumonic infiltrates. The majority of patients recover spontaneously.
   B. **Chronic pulmonary infection**. In less than 2% of patients, the primary pulmonary infection evolves into a chronic process.
   C. **Chronic infection of other organ systems**
      1. Chronic extrapulmonary foci of C. immitis infection may follow early dissemination. The most frequent foci are abscesses and sinus tract formation of the musculoskeletal system and lytic bone lesions, especially involving the spine.
      2. Meningitis is the most life-threatening complication of chronic extrapulmonary coccidioidomycosis, manifesting as headache, fever, altered mental status, cranial nerve palsies, and other neurologic deficits.
   D. **Disseminated disease in the immunocompromised host.** Impairment of T cell-mediated immune function is associated with a significant risk of disseminated infection with C. immitis. Chest radiographs usually show a bilateral diffuse reticulonodular picture. Patients with advanced HIV disease, particularly those with CD4+ counts less than 200 cells/μL are at increased risk for progressive disseminated C. immitis infection.

II. **Diagnosis**
   A. Laboratory diagnosis is by culture, biopsy, serologic test for coccidioidal IgM antibodies in serum or CSF or by detection of rising titer of coccidioidal IgG. The fungus can be cultured from blood or tissue in 3 to 5 days. In pulmonary disease, it is possible to detect the fungus in sputum smears or cultures, but detection may require bronchoalveolar lavage or transbronchial biopsy. CSF cultures are positive in 50% of patients with meningitis.
   B. Skin testing is not useful because the skin test result remains positive long after acute infection has subsided, and it is negative for many patients with underlying immunodeficiency and disseminated coccidioidomycosis.

III. **Treatment**
   A. Acutely ill patients with disseminated disease should be treated with amphotericin B, 1.0 to 1.5 mg/kg/day IV for a cumulative dose of 1.0 to 2.5 g. Once the acute disease is controlled, life-long suppressive therapy with ketoconazole (400 mg per day orally) or fluconazole (Diflucan) (400 to 600 mg per day orally) should be initiated to prevent relapses.
   B. Fluconazole (Diflucan) (800 mg per day orally) is the recommended

initial treatment in patients with coccidioidal meningitis. Itraconazole (Sporanox), 300 mg twice daily for 3 days and then 200 mg twice daily for 12 weeks, may also be effective. Intrathecal amphotericin B should be considered in patients who do not respond clinically after 1 to 2 months of therapy. §

References: See page 81.

Mycobacterium Avium Complex

Mycobacterium avium complex (MAC) is ubiquitous in the environment. In patients with AIDS it is one of the most common serious opportunistic infections.

I. **Clinical presentation**
    A. Disseminated MAC infection usually occurs in AIDS patients with a CD4 count of <50 cells/μL. Symptoms include persistent fever, night sweats, fatigue, weight loss, anorexia, abdominal pain, and chronic diarrhea.
    B. Hepatosplenomegaly, lymphadenopathy, and (rarely) jaundice also may be present. Anemia is the most common laboratory abnormality, and leukopenia, elevated alkaline phosphatase levels, or low albumin may also occur.

II. **Diagnosis**. Mycobacterial culture of peripheral blood is sensitive for disseminated MAC infection. Mycobacterial blood culture establishes the diagnosis in 86 to 98% of cases. One blood culture identifies 91% of patients with MAC bacteremia; a second blood culture increases the identification rate to 98%. Culture of bone marrow, lymph node or liver is sensitive than blood culture.

III. **Treatment of disseminated MAC infection.** Treatment should begin with clarithromycin (Biaxin), 500 mg twice daily, plus ethambutol (approximately 15 mg/kg/day). Rifabutin may be added. Treatment should be continued indefinitely.

IV. **Prophylaxis**. Patients with <50 CD4 lymphocytes/μl who exhibit no clinical evidence of active mycobacterial disease should receive prophylaxis with either clarithromycin (Biaxin), 500 mg twice daily, or azithromycin (Zithromax), 1200 mg (2 tabs) weekly; the latter could be administered with rifabutin (Mycobutin) 300 mg daily.

References: See page 81.

Kaposi's Sarcoma

Kaposi's sarcoma (KS) is the most common neoplasm affecting HIV-infected individuals. The risk of developing KS is greatest in the homosexual male population (up to 73,000 fold risk). Highly-active antiretroviral therapy has brought about a 61% decline in the incidence of KS.

I. **Pathogenesis.** Kaposi's sarcoma herpesvirus (KSHV) is present in peripheral blood mononuclear cells from patients with HIV-KS and predicts subsequent development of KS. The virus is sexually transmitted.

II. **Clinical Presentation**
   A. KS presents as palpable, firm, non-tender, cutaneous nodules, ranging from .5 to 2 cm in diameter. Early, non-palpable lesions resembling small ecchymoses may be observed.
   B. Lesions may appear as small raised plaques, nodules or large bulky plaques. Lesions are typically violaceous in light-skinned individuals, but may appear brown or black in dark-skinned individuals. Oral lesions are common and may be the first site of disease. Progression is frequently observed in the setting of acute opportunistic infection.
   C. **Visceral disease**
      1. **Gastrointestinal KS** is the most common presentation of visceral disease, and it may be present in up to 40% of patients at diagnosis. Symptoms such as bleeding, perforation and obstruction are uncommon.
      2. **Pulmonary KS** presents with dyspnea, cough or bronchospasm. Disease may be difficult to distinguish from an infectious process. Death due to respiratory failure is common. The chest X-ray typically shows a reticular-nodular pattern and pleural effusion is often present (40-50%). Diagnosis is based upon visual documentation of characteristic endobronchial lesions. Gallium scanning may be help to rule-out pulmonary opportunistic infection.

III. **Cutaneous complications of KS**
   A. Pain or discomfort may occur as lesions progress at any site. Edema of the lower extremity and facial edema may occur. Cellulitis may develop in areas that are extensively involved with KS, particularly if edema is present.
   B. A biopsy is generally recommended to diagnose KS. The differential diagnosis of KS includes bacillary angiomatosis, cutaneous mycobacterial disease, cutaneous fungal disease, and angiosarcoma.

IV. **Treatment of Kaposi's sarcoma**
   A. **Local therapy** is appropriate for symptomatic local involvement or small lesions which are cosmetically unsightly.
      1. **Radiotherapy** is effective for facial edema and lower extremity edema, but it is less effective than chemotherapy.
      2. **Intralesional vinblastine**, 0.01 mg vinblastine in 0.1 mL sterile water per lesion, is useful for small, cosmetically unsightly lesions. Repeated treatments may be necessary. This treatment
      3. **Cryotherapy** with liquid nitrogen is effective for small cosmetically unsightly lesions.
   B. **Systemic chemotherapy** is indicated for widespread symptomatic disease, rapidly progressive disease and visceral disease.
      1. **Liposomal anthracyclines** are first-line therapy for advanced cutaneous or visceral disease. Liposomal preparations of doxorubicin

and daunorubicin are highly effective.

2. **The doxorubicin, bleomycin, vincristine (ABV)** regimen is less commonly employed for patients with advanced symptomatic disease and is more toxic than the liposomal agents.

3. **Paclitaxel (Taxol)** is a highly active agent used as second-line therapy in patients refractory initial therapy.

Single AgentSystemic Therapy for Kaposi's Sarcoma

Agent	Dose	Response	Recommended Use
Vincristine	2 mg/wk	20-59%	Rarely used alone, non-myelosuppressive
Vinblastine	0.5-1 mg/kg/wk	25-30%	Rarely used alone
Etoposide	50 mg po qd, alternate weeks or 150 mg/m^2 IV qd for 3d q3-4 wks	36-75%	As single agent for prior treatment failure
Adriamycin	20 mg/m^2 every other week	53%	Rarely used alone
Bleomycin	10-15 u/m^2 q2wks or 20 mg/m^2/d x 3d	65%	Nonmyelosuppressive; use if intolerance to other agents
Paclitaxel	100 mg/m^2 q2 wks	53%	Treatment failures
Liposomal Doxorubicin	20 mg/m^2 q2-3 wks	45-74%	Single agent
Liposomal Daunorubicin	40 mg/m^2 q2 wks	28-55 %	Single agent First line therapy
Vinorelbine	30 mg/m^2 q 2 wks	40%	Treatment Failures

Combination Chemotherapy

Agents	Dose	Response	Recommended Use
Vincristine/ Vinblastine	2 mg 0.1 mg/kg alternate weeks	45 %	Diffuse, disease, minimally symptomatic
Adriamycin/ Bleomycin/ Vincristine	10-20 mg/m^2 10 mg/m^2 q 14d 2 mg	87%	Diffuse symptomatic disease, edema, rapid response desired
Bleomycin/	10 mg/m^2 q 14d		Diffuse disease, symptomatic,

Vincristine	2 mg		patients with neutropenia or poor bone marrow reserve

C. Interferon-alpha
   1. Interferon therapy requires some level of intact immune function to achieve a response.
   2. Combination therapy with low-dose interferon (3-18 million units/day, 5 days/week) and standard dose zidovudine or didanosine is effective and is associated with less drug-induced toxicity.

Interferon-Alpha

Agent	Dose	Response	Recommended Use
alpha-interferon	3-18 mu/d 5 d/wk	30-40%	Diffuse progressive disease, but with no or minimal symptoms, use with antiviral therapy and a CD4 $>100/mm^3$

Therapeutic Recommendations

Minimal disease Stable or slowly progressive	1. Combination antiretroviral therapy 2. Alpha-interferon
Minimal disease Rapidly progressive or extensive asymptomatic	1. Combination antiretroviral therapy 2. Alpha-interferon with antiretroviral therapy if CD4 $>100/mm^3$ 3. Liposomal anthracycline
Widespread symptomatic	1. Liposomal anthracyclenes 2. Adriamycin, bleomycin, vincristine (ABV)
Locally symptomatic	1. Radiotherapy 2. Laser (oral lesions)
Local cosmesis	1. Intralesional chemotherapy 2. Radiotherapy 3. Cryotherapy
Cytopenic patients	1. Vincristine and/or 2. Bleomycin 3. Use G- or GM-CSF

Refractory disease	1. Paclitaxel 2. Vinorelbine

References: See page 81.

HIV-Associated Lymphoma

HIV-associated, non-Hodgkin's lymphoma occurs in 5-10% of individuals with HIV infection. The incidence of lymphoma in this population has been rising and may reflect prolonged survival related to the use of highly-active antiretroviral therapy and infection prophylaxis.

I. **Pathophysiology**
   A. HIV-associated non-Hodgkin's lymphomas are virtually all of B-cell origin. Most are intermediate- or high-grade lymphomas categorized as large cell (60%) or small non-cleaved lymphomas (25%).
   B. Seventy-five percent of patients with systemic lymphoma have a CD4 cell count>50/mm^3. Most present with extranodal disease, often in the bone marrow, meninges, liver or GI tract.

Comparison of Molecular and Clinical Features of AIDS-lymphomas

	Systemic	CNS	Primary Effusion
Histology	Large Cell (60%) Small noncleaved (30%)	Large Cell	Pleomorphic large cell
Clonality	Monoclonal polyclonal	Monoclonal	Monoclonal
EBV	Present in minority	Always present	Often present
HIV-8	Absent	Absent	Present
Median CD4+	100	30	90
Survival (median)	6-8 months	3 months	5 months

II. **Treatment**
   A. Complete response occurs in 33-62% of patients. Relapse occurs in 25% of complete responders within 6 months. Median survival is 4-8 months, with about half dying of lymphoma and half of opportunistic infection. Median survivals as long as 18 months have been reported.
   B. Low-dose mBACOD is associated with a similar response and survival as standard treatment regimens.

Low-dose mBACOD		
Agent	**Dose**	**Days**
Cyclophosphamide	300 mg/m^2, IV	1
Doxorubicin	25 mg/m^2, IV	1
Bleomycin	4 mg/m^2, IV	1
Vincristine	2 mg, IV	1
Dexamethasone	3 mg/m^2, po	1-5
Methotrexate	500 mg/m^2, IV Folinic acid rescue 25 mg q 6h x 6 beginning 24hours after completion of MTX	15

C. **Aggressive chemotherapy** is associated with a higher risk of death due to opportunistic infection Myeloid growth factors (G-CSF, GM-CSF) have been shown to reduce hematologic toxicity in patients receiving standard-dose chemotherapy. Myeloid growth factors are usually not needed in patients receiving a reduced-dose treatment regimen.

CHOP chemotherapy		
Agent	**Dose**	**Day**
Cyclophosphamide	750 mg/m^2, IV	1
Doxorubicin	40 mg/m^2, IV	1
Vincristine	2 mg	1
Prednisone	100 mg, IV	1-5
G- or GM-CSF	5 mg/kg/day	4-13 of each treatment cycle

D. Meningeal prophylaxis with intrathecal MTX or cytosine arabinoside is indicated for patients with a positive bone marrow biopsy, small noncleaved histology, paranasal or epidural involvement, and for advanced stage IV disease. The dosage of intrathecal cytosine arabinoside is 50 mg in 6 cc preservative-free saline, weekly, during the first four weeks of therapy. Pneumocystis carinii prophylaxis with trimethoprim-sulfamethoxazole, dapsone, or inhaled pentamidine is also recommended.

E. Treatment recommendations: Systemic non-Hodgkin's lymphoma
  1. **All patients with CD4 <100/mm^3**: Low-dose chemotherapy
  2. **CD4 >100/mm^3**: Consider standard-dose chemotherapy in selected patients.
  3. **Antibiotic prophylaxis** for P. carinii in all patients.
  4. **Meningeal prophylaxis** for those with small noncleaved histology, bone marrow involvement, paranasal sinus involvement, or epidural disease.
  5. **Antiviral therapy:**
     a. Combination antiviral therapy should be continued with chemotherapy
     b. Zidovudine is not recommended due to risk of overlapping myelosuppression.

III. Primary central nervous system lymphoma in HIV infection
  A. These individuals present with severe immunodeficiency, most with CD4 lymphocyte counts <50/mm^3. Antitoxoplasma therapy is appropriate only in those individuals who are toxoplasma seropositive. Patients who are seronegative should undergo brain biopsy to rule out the presence of lymphoma.
   1. Solitary lesions are more likely to be lymphoma.
   2. Up to 20% have a positive CSF cytology. A lumbar puncture should be performed if not contraindicated.
   3. Thallium-SPECT is usually positive in lymphoma, and it is usually negative in toxoplasmosis.
   4. PCR for EBV in CSF: 80-85% sensitive, 90% specific for lymphoma. PCR testing may reduce the need for invasive diagnosis.
  B. Treatment consists of whole brain radiotherapy. Three quarters of these individuals will have a clinical responses to therapy (improvement in neurologic symptoms). The median survival is only 2-4 months, and most deaths are caused by opportunistic infections. §

References

References may be obtained via the internet at www.ccspublishing.com.

Index

Titles from Current Clinical Strategies Publishing

In Bookstores Worldwide

Medicine, 1998 Edition

Pediatrics 5 Minute Review, 1998-99 Edition

Anesthesiology, 1999-2000 Edition

Handbook of Psychiatric Drugs, 1998-99 Edition

Gynecology and Obstetrics, 1999-2000 Edition

Manual of HIV/AIDS Therapy, 2001 Edition

Family Medicine, 2000 Edition

Practice Parameters in Medicine and Primary Care, 1999-2000 Edition

Surgery, 1999-2000 Edition

Pediatric Drug Reference, 2000 Edition

Critical Care Medicine, 2000 Edition

Outpatient Medicine, 1997 Edition

History and Physical Examination in Medicine, 2001-2002 Edition

Psychiatry, 1999-2000 Edition

Pediatrics, 2000 Edition

Physicians' Drug Resource, 1999 Edition

CD-ROM and Softcover Book

Internet Journals from
Current Clinical Strategies Publishing

Journal of Primary Care Medicine
Journal of Medicine
Journal of Pediatric Medicine
Journal of Surgery
Journal of Family Medicine
Journal of Emergency Medicine and Acute Primary
Care
Journal of Psychiatry
Journal of AIDS/HIV

---

www.ccspublishing.com